CHILDHOOD OBESITY

CAUSES, MANAGEMENT AND CHALLENGES

D0898301

CHILDREN'S ISSUES, LAWS AND PROGRAMS

Additional books in this series can be found on Nova's website under the Series tab.

Additional e-books in this series can be found on Nova's website under the e-book tab.

CHILDHOOD OBESITY

CAUSES, MANAGEMENT AND CHALLENGES

CALLUM G. JACKSON
EDITOR

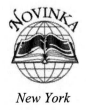

New York

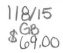

NOTICE TO THE READER

The Publisher has taken reasonable care in the preparation of this book, but makes no expressed or implied warranty of any kind and assumes no responsibility for any errors or omissions. No liability is assumed for incidental or consequential damages in connection with or arising out of information contained in this book. The Publisher shall not be liable for any special, consequential, or exemplary damages resulting, in whole or in part, from the readers' use of, or reliance upon, this material. Any parts of this book based on government reports are so indicated and copyright is claimed for those parts to the extent applicable to compilations of such works.

Independent verification should be sought for any data, advice or recommendations contained in this book. In addition, no responsibility is assumed by the publisher for any injury and/or damage to persons or property arising from any methods, products, instructions, ideas or otherwise contained in this publication.

This publication is designed to provide accurate and authoritative information with regard to the subject matter covered herein. It is sold with the clear understanding that the Publisher is not engaged in rendering legal or any other professional services. If legal or any other expert assistance is required, the services of a competent person should be sought. FROM A DECLARATION OF PARTICIPANTS JOINTLY ADOPTED BY A COMMITTEE OF THE AMERICAN BAR ASSOCIATION AND A COMMITTEE OF PUBLISHERS.

Additional color graphics may be available in the e-book version of this book.

Library of Congress Cataloging-in-Publication Data

ISBN: 978-1-62618-874-7

Library of Congress Control Number: 2013938113

Published by Nova Science Publishers, Inc. † New York

CONTENTS

PREFACE

In this book, the authors present current research in the study of the causes, management and challenges in childhood obesity. Topics discussed include the genomics of childhood obesity and obesity-related disorders; the cardiometabolic impact of childhood obesity and the potential role of exercise; contributory influences promoting childhood adiposity in a Mediterranean island population; and an observation of obesity and mental health in the young.

Chapter 1 – The genomics of childhood obesity is an important topic to investigate and gain a better understanding of the role of genes and abnormalities which account for about 50% of obesity. Genotyping, chromosomal microarrays, genome-wide association studies (GWAS) and next generation sequencing are methods used to identify genes and defects in obesity-related syndromes and obesity. The authors' current understanding of genetic factors contributing to childhood obesity will be addressed along with the latest developments in diet and gene interaction, structural chromosomal anomalies, mutations and polymorphisms, epigenetics and discussion of obesity-related syndromes.

Obesity is a global health problem which is on the rise due to sedentary lifestyles, over-nutrition and to a great extent genetic factors and susceptibility. The prevalence of childhood overweight and obesity has doubled over the past 30 years. At least, nine genetic loci have been identified to directly cause non-syndromic obesity while 58 loci are known to contribute. More than 150 loss-of-function coding mutations have been associated with monogenic obesity (e.g., *MC4R*, the most commonly recognized single gene causing childhood obesity and found in about 4% of cases). Rare and common DNA variants are also associated with obesity but yet most obesity genes are yet to be discovered. Studies have shown that the childhood obesity epidemic is due to multi-factorial causes including the interaction of genes and the environment such as diet with GWAS showing an interaction of individual nutritional components with increased weight. High heritability estimates for obesity also indicate the presence of causative genes and genomic regions including structural chromosomal abnormalities (e.g., 3p25 duplications, 10q22.3-23.2 and 16p11.2 deletions). Genetic changes are not solely responsible for the increased prevalence as mutations are not accumulating at the rate required to account for such an increase. Thus, an obesogenic environment is most likely due to complex and undefined gene-diet and gene-physical activity interactions.

One of the most classical genetic obesity disorders is Prader-Willi syndrome (PWS), a complex genomic imprinting neurodevelopmental disorder with loss of paternally expressed genes from the chromosome 15q11-q13 region. PWS is characterized by hypotonia, a poor suck, hypogonadism /hypogenitalism, growth hormone deficiency with short stature, small hands and feet, learning/behavioral problems and hyperphagia leading to early childhood obesity. A second genetic condition with obesity as a major feature is the fragile X syndrome, the most common cause of familial intellectual disability. Physical features include an elongated face, prominent ears, and post-pubertal macroorchidism. Severe obesity is often associated with a Prader-Willi phenotype including hyperphagia, lack of satiation and hypogonadism with delayed puberty. A third obesity-related genetic disorder is Alström syndrome, a rare autosomal recessive condition with characteristic vision and hearing deficits, truncal obesity with insulin resistance, type 2 diabetes, hypertriglyceridemia, short stature and cardiovascular, hepatic, and renal dysfunction. This syndrome is caused by a ciliary protein abnormality which is in common with Bardet-Biedl syndrome, another single gene condition with obesity as a major manifestation. Alström syndrome provides an example into the pathogenic mechanisms underlying obesity and diabetes leading to potentially important insights into ciliopathies as causes of obesity and diabetes, conditions common in the general population.

Chapter 2 – Obesity in children is a significant public health problem in the United States as the number of adolescents who are overweight has tripled in the last 30 years so that 17% (or 12.5 million) of children and adolescents aged 2—19 years are now classified as obese based on body mass index (BMI). Excess weight in adolescence frequently persists into young adulthood, and has a strong adverse cardiometabolic impact. Additionally, available data suggest that children may be living increasingly sedentary lifestyles, which may exacerbate the effects of obesity on health and function, both now and in the future. Therefore there is currently a need to understand the causes and consequences of childhood obesity and to develop effective intervention approaches to prevent its development and/or the pathological effects of obesity. The purpose of this review is to provide an integrated examination of how obesity affects the risk for cardiovascular and metabolic (diabetes and bone) diseases, with emphasis on the role of physical exercise as a prevention and treatment strategy. For example, atherosclerosis starts in childhood and obesity appears to accelerate the development of atherosclerotic lesions. It has also been shown that childhood obesity clusters with components of the metabolic syndrome, such as high concentration of low-density lipoprotein (LDL), low concentration of high-density lipoprotein (HDL), insulin resistance and hypertension. Obesity is also a major risk factor for pre-diabetes and type 2 diabetes (T2DM). In obese people, fasting and postprandial plasma glucose concentration are the best clinical predictors for the progression from insulin resistance to T2DM The glycemic control also determines the future risk of micro and macro vascular complications, which demonstrates the inter-connection between metabolic and cardiovascular systems. Understanding how obesity affects bone health in children has become increasingly important. Many of the available studies that have assessed the effect of childhood obesity on bone accrual have resulted in conflicting results. However, recent evidence has shown that bone is a metabolically active tissue that responds to hormones like insulin, and produces proteins that affect pancreatic and adipose tissues, and that these communication processes are disrupted in the presence of obesity. Thus, obesity has integrated effects on multiple organs and tissues. Since physical exercise promotes bone loading, stimulates better glycemic control, and has protective effects on lipid profile and the cardiovascular system, an important focus of the authors' research and this review is on the potential benefits of exercise for improving the health of obese children.

Chapter 3 – The Maltese population is a small island population in the Central Mediterranean. The nutritional concerns relating to Maltese children in the mid-twentieth century were primarily those relating to undernutrition and insufficient body weight when compared to their British counterparts. There has been in the last decades a shift in the childhood weight concerns with the observation of an alarming rise in childhood adiposity reaching to 28.8% and 32.7% in 5-year old body and girls respectively; and 48.9% and 45.1% respectively at 9 years of age.

The underlying cause for this rise has been shown to be partly related to perinatal and early childhood feeding programming that appears to offset any later attempts to control for later childhood adiposity. A further association has been described for childhood adiposity to an increased mean passive activity time with a corresponding negative association to mean active physical activity and sleeping times. Transgenerational associations towards a familiar tendency to adiposity have been observed these possibly being related to the family's socio-economic status or a family history of metabolic syndrome components. It is advised that parents of children at risk – low or high birth weight; bottle fed children; early childhood obesity – should be regularly advised actively regarding health lifestyle and nutrition options. The observed relationship between childhood adiposity to the combination of decreased physical activity and increased energy-dense foods suggests that life-style intervention could have a possible positive influence in decreasing the problems of childhood adiposity.

Chapter 4 – Obesity is getting to be amore prevailing disease all over the world. It is estimated that nearly 250 millions of obese and overweight persons in the world. In the last three decades childhood obesity also got prevalent as high as 18-30% in developed countries as USA, Italy, Germany and England. Also in the developing countries, obesity is increasing, according to the data collected by WHO from 94 countries. The mean prevalence of obesity is 3.3% in these countries. In African and Asian countries under weight is 2.5-3.5 times more prevalent than obesity.

It is well known that the risk of developing hypertension insulin resistance and hyper insulinemia are high in the obese persons. Obesity is also an independent risk factor in coronary heart disease, childhood obesity also has been shown to be having such negative effects on health, such as hypertension, abnormal glucose tolerance, x-syndrome and cardiovascular disease. Development of obesity is affected by many factors such as genetic, family history, lack of physical activity, gender, income and nutritional habits of fatty meals consumption.

Chapter 5 – In the last decade or so there has been an increasing awareness of the association between weight changes, mental health and psychotropic medications. The relationship is rather complex with changes in weight occurring as part of many psychiatric conditions including depression, eating disorders, ADHD, anxiety disorders and also just as part of stressful periods for an individual.

The relationship gets more complex with medications especially Second Generation Antipsychotics (SGAs) used in the treatment of psychoses. There is a clear association with the use of medications, weight gain and medical morbidity. A big need of the hour is to look at pragmatic and informed approaches to intervention in these situations when weight gain becomes a commonly encountered accompaniment of psychiatric treatment. A preventive and early intervention focus is critical in the comprehensive management to avoid physical co-morbidity. This clinical review attempts to address some of these issues with a specific focus on metabolic syndrome.

In: Childhood Obesity
Editor: Callum G. Jackson

ISBN: 978-1-62618-874-7
© 2013 Nova Science Publishers, Inc.

Chapter 1

GENOMICS OF CHILDHOOD OBESITY AND OBESITY-RELATED DISORDERS

Merlin G. Butler[*]

Departments of Psychiatry & Behavioral Sciences and Pediatrics
Kansas University Medical Center, Kansas City, Kansas, US

ABSTRACT

The genomics of childhood obesity is an important topic to investigate and gain a better understanding of the role of genes and abnormalities which account for about 50% of obesity. Genotyping, chromosomal microarrays, genome-wide association studies (GWAS) and next generation sequencing are methods used to identify genes and defects in obesity-related syndromes and obesity. Our current understanding of genetic factors contributing to childhood obesity will be addressed along with the latest developments in diet and gene interaction, structural chromosomal anomalies, mutations and polymorphisms, epigenetics and discussion of obesity-related syndromes.

Obesity is a global health problem which is on the rise due to sedentary lifestyles, over-nutrition and to a great extent genetic factors and susceptibility. The prevalence of childhood overweight and obesity has doubled over the past 30 years. At least, nine genetic loci have been

[*] Correspondence to: Merlin G. Butler, M.D., Ph.D., F.F.A.C.M.G., Department of Psychiatry & Behavioral Sciences and Pediatrics, Kansas University Medical Center, Kansas City, Kansas, 3901 Rainbow Boulevard, MS4015, Kansas City, KS 66160. Phone: (913) 588-1873, Fax: (913) 588-1305, E-mail: mbutler4@kumc.edu.

identified to directly cause non-syndromic obesity while 58 loci are known to contribute. More than 150 loss-of-function coding mutations have been associated with monogenic obesity (e.g., *MC4R*, the most commonly recognized single gene causing childhood obesity and found in about 4% of cases). Rare and common DNA variants are also associated with obesity but yet most obesity genes are yet to be discovered. Studies have shown that the childhood obesity epidemic is due to multi-factorial causes including the interaction of genes and the environment such as diet with GWAS showing an interaction of individual nutritional components with increased weight. High heritability estimates for obesity also indicate the presence of causative genes and genomic regions including structural chromosomal abnormalities (e.g., 3p25 duplications, 10q22.3-23.2 and 16p11.2 deletions). Genetic changes are not solely responsible for the increased prevalence as mutations are not accumulating at the rate required to account for such an increase. Thus, an obesogenic environment is most likely due to complex and undefined gene-diet and gene-physical activity interactions.

One of the most classical genetic obesity disorders is Prader-Willi syndrome (PWS), a complex genomic imprinting neurodevelopmental disorder with loss of paternally expressed genes from the chromosome 15q11-q13 region. PWS is characterized by hypotonia, a poor suck, hypogonadism/hypogenitalism, growth hormone deficiency with short stature, small hands and feet, learning/behavioral problems and hyperphagia leading to early childhood obesity. A second genetic condition with obesity as a major feature is the fragile X syndrome, the most common cause of familial intellectual disability. Physical features include an elongated face, prominent ears, and post-pubertal macroorchidism. Severe obesity is often associated with a Prader-Willi phenotype including hyperphagia, lack of satiation and hypogonadism with delayed puberty. A third obesity-related genetic disorder is Alström syndrome, a rare autosomal recessive condition with characteristic vision and hearing deficits, truncal obesity with insulin resistance, type 2 diabetes, hypertriglyceridemia, short stature and cardiovascular, hepatic, and renal dysfunction. This syndrome is caused by a ciliary protein abnormality which is in common with Bardet-Biedl syndrome, another single gene condition with obesity as a major manifestation. Alström syndrome provides an example into the pathogenic mechanisms underlying obesity and diabetes leading to potentially important insights into ciliopathies as causes of obesity and diabetes, conditions common in the general population.

INTRODUCTION

Obesity is one of the most pressing global health problems affecting each continent worldwide and leading to several co-morbidities including diabetes, mellitus, heart disease and fatty liver, sleep apnea, musculo-skeletal disorders, hypertension and also cancer [1-3]. Although the prevalence of obesity and diabetes are heritable traits, the susceptibility to obesity by genetic factors alone cannot account for the increased prevalence during the past two to three decades. An obesity-promoting environment and major societal changes such as a sedentary lifestyle and over-nutrition do exist in both children and adults and impose a substantial economic burden. Since the 1980s, the mean body mass index (BMI) in humans has increased throughout the world by 0.4-0.5 kg/m^2 per decade in adults [3]. Over 10% of all adults worldwide are classified as having obesity (BMI $\geq$ 30 kg/m2) while childhood overweight and obesity prevalence worldwide has increased from 4.2% in 1990 to 6.7% in 2010 and is expected to continue to increase [3-4]. Increased weight gain during infancy does correlate with the findings of obesity in adulthood leading to obesity-associated disorders and a shortened life expectancy. Behind this epidemic is the role of genetic factors including major single genes and minor genomic variants and polymorphisms impacting on gene function [1,5,6]. This chapter will focus on genetics and gene mechanisms along with rare or uncommon known genetic syndromes having obesity as a key feature with emphasis on the genomics of childhood obesity.

With the advent of new and varied genetic techniques including high resolution chromosome analysis, fluorescence *in situ* hybridization (FISH) with single DNA probes, structural DNA microarray hybridization with copy number variant and single nucleotide polymorphism (SNP) probes and next generation sequencing, structural chromosomal and DNA abnormalities have been identified involving genomic regions where genes causing obesity are located or linked to obesity traits. The genetic obesity-based research has led to a review in 2006 of 176 gene mutations in 11 different single genes, 50 loci related to known single gene conditions with obesity, 244 adiposity related genes (in mice), 408 animal model-based obesity traits and 253 quantitative obesity traits in humans [7-9] and increased numbers since that time. The following includes a list of reported chromosome abnormalities (deletions and/or duplications) in humans with syndromic obesity excluding Prader-Willi syndrome, the most common known cause of morbid obesity in children and will be discussed later: chromosome 1p36 deletion; chromosome 2q37.3 deletion; chromosome 3p23 duplication; 3p25.3 duplication (contains the

GHRL gene); chromosome 4q32.1 duplication; 4q35.1 duplication; chromosome 5p13.1 duplication; chromosome 6q16.2 deletion (*SIM1* gene); 6q22.2 deletion; 6q24.3 duplication; 6q15-q21 deletion (*SIM1* gene); 6q16-q21 deletion (*SIM1* gene); 6q16.1-q16.3 deletion (*SIM1* gene); chromosome 7q36 deletion; chromosome 9p23 deletion; 9q34 deletion; 9q34.3 deletion; 9q33.3q34 duplication; chromosome 10q22.3q23.2 duplication; chromosome 11p12-p14 deletion; 11p13-p14.2 deletion (*BDNF* gene); 11p11.2 deletion; chromosome 12p13.1 duplication; 12qter deletion; chromosome 14q32.2 hypomethylation status (maternal disomy 14); chromosome 16q13 duplication, 16p11.2 deletion (*SH2B1* gene); 16q11.2-q13 duplication (*FTO* gene); chromosome 18q12.2-q21.1 deletion; chromosome 19q12-q13.2 duplication; 19q13.2 deletion; chromosome 20q13.13-q13.32 deletion; chromosome 22q11.2 deletion; chromosome Xq26.3-q27.3 deletion (*FMR1* gene); Xq23q25 duplication; Xp11.3p21.1 duplication; Xp11.4q11.2 inversion; and Xq27.1-q28 deletion (FMR1 gene) [9]. Genomic scanning methods have also led to the discovery of genetic differences as important findings among humans with obesity and referred to as copy number or structural variants (CNVs). For example, small deletions of chromosome 16p11.2 band have been reported in about 0.5-0.7% of individuals with severe obesity including the *SH2B1* gene which modulates leptin sensitivity in humans and involved with caloric intake and regulation [10-12]. Studies have also shown that rare CNVs greater than 2 Mb in size were present in 1.3% of obese humans and absent in lean controls with the CNVs disrupting candidate genes for obesity such as the *UCP1* gene. With reported structural chromosomal abnormities and candidate obesity genes located in the abnormal cytogenetic regions, the search for additional genes and genomic variants have continued including heritability studies to determine the influence of genetic factors for obesity in monozygotic and dizygotic twins. At least, 58 gene loci have been reported to contribute to obesity due to multiple genes (polygenic) causes [2].

Strong genetic influences do impact on the percentage of body fat in humans, as well as, waist circumference, degree of physical activity, energy expenditure and eating behavior with heritability for body mass index in adults estimated at 40-70% [13,14]. Genetic factors also account for a high BMI in children estimated at about 80% of cases with mutations in specific genes found for 5-10% of childhood obesity [14-17]. The definition of heritability is the proportion of the variation seen in the phenotype due to genetic causes among individuals studied [18]. Adoption studies show that when monozygotic twins are reared apart or together, they have a very similar correlation value at about 0.7 for their BMI status. For dizygotic twins reared apart the correlations average to about 0.2 and for dizygotic twins reared together the correlations average to about 0.3 [19-21]. Therefore, genetic influences on BMI are supported by these studies but increased physical activity and exercise can lower the influence of genes on BMI and the level of obesity. Ethnicity may also impact on the genetic predisposition for obesity.

Single gene disorders such as monogenic forms of obesity have been found for loss of function mutations in at least five recessive genes including *LEP, LEPR, POMC, PCSK1* and *MC4R* and nine separate loci. When these five recessive genes are inactivated then severe hyperphagia and early-onset of extreme obesity results in humans. Additional features are also seen in those having recessive forms of obesity including congenital leptin deficiency and alterations in the immune system with frequent childhood infections and delayed puberty due to underdevelopment of the sex organs [15,22-24].

Those individuals with *POMC* gene deficiency can present with hypoadrenalism secondary to low ACTH levels and hypoglycemia, jaundice and even neonatal death. They also may have pale skin and red hair color in Caucasians due to impairment in pigment production. Those with *PCSK1* gene deficiencies are prone to having hypoglycemia and other endocrine-related problems. Individuals with complete *MC4R* deficiency can also have increased lean mass and bone mineral density with tall stature. *MC4R* deficiency is the most common cause of single gene or monogenic obesity in humans and heterozygotes can also be affected indicating some degree of dominance, a prevalence of 1-2.5% in people with a BMI greater than 30 [25,26]. There are over 150 loss-of-function coding mutations of the *MC4R* gene associated with obesity while two gain-of-function polymorphisms are associated with protection from obesity. Thus, the vast majority of variants of the *MC4R* gene impact on obesity with a single recognized variant (SNP re17782313) associated with increased hunger, snacking and caloric intake and decreased satiety [15].

Advanced genome-wide association studies (GWAS) have found strong associations with the Fat mass and obesity associated (*FTO*) gene locus and BMI with an additional 35 SNPs in 33 loci [27,28]. Intron 1 of the *FTO* gene is thought to be the major genetic contributor to polygenic obesity in populations from European ancestry. About 1 in 5 adults of European ancestry are homozygous for the risk allele of the *FTO* gene and they weigh about 3 kilograms more with a 1.7-fold increased odds of developing obesity when compared with those individuals not inheriting a risk allele for this gene [28]. Complete absence of FTO gene expression in humans is lethal and thus essential for normal central nervous and cardiovascular system development.

Of the nine loci associated with extreme obesity identified so far at the genome-wide level, five (i.e., *FTO, MC4R, TMEM18, MSRA, NPC1*) are known to influence a high BMI and a large waist circumference [25,29-32]. Four other loci (i.e., *MAF, PTER, PRL, SDCCAG8*) are more specific for increasing measures of extreme obesity with overlapping evidence in both children and adults [32]. Several obesity-related genes (i.e., *FTO, MC4R, POMC, SH2B1, BDNF, NPC1, NRXN3* and *NEGR1*) identified through GWAS studies have been found to be highly expressed in the central nervous system indicating a key for regulation of food intake and monogenic causes of human obesity [33-35]. There may also be differences in association with obesity depending on sex specifically for Chinese children and variants in some of these genes [35]. GWAS analyses also investigated other obesity measures including body fat distribution, waist circumference or waist to hip ratio and their relationship to each gene loci. Five loci (i.e., *FTO, MC4R, NRXN3, TFAP2B, MSRA*) which have found to be only associated with BMI as a measure of obesity [36]. Studies have also shown a CNV and SNP-based whole-genome analysis identified a 45-kb deletion near the *NEGR1* and *GPRC5BT* genes and associated with variation in BMI.

A recent genome-wide association meta-analysis has identified new extreme childhood obesity loci for *OLFM4* at 13q14 and *HOXB5* at 17q21 [37]. Two ethnic specific polymorphisms in the *AGRP* gene has also been examined in relationship to nutrient and energy parameters. In whites, a smaller proportion of total energy was derived from fat for the Ala67Thr heterozygotes with a lower intake of fats and increased level of carbohydrate consumption. In blacks, greater protein intake was associated with the -38C > T promoter polymorphism [38]. Additionally, the *LY86* gene was associated with waist to hip ratio and a common CNV found on chromosome 10p11.22 was associated with BMI in a Chinese population study covering four genes; one of the genes (*PPYR1*) may be an obesity candidate gene [34]. There are now at least 61 common gene variants reported in at least 58 loci that have been associated with an obesity phenotype using genome-wide studies and meeting statistical significance but yet these results show only a small percentage of the many genes to be discovered that play a role in the causation of obesity [15] (Table 1).

Table 1. List of obesity gene regions or loci and their description with obesity phenotype

Regions/description	Gene or chromosome location
Loci identified by genome-wide studies (GWAS, linkage, CNV/SNP microarrays) associated with child and/or adult BMI and including extreme obesity	FTO; TMEM18; GNPDA2; INSIG2; MC4R; NEGR1; BDNF; KCTD15; PCSK; CTNNBL1; MTCH2; NPC1; MAF; PTER; PRL; FAIM2; TFAP2B; SEC16B; ETV5; AIF1; GPRL5BB; MAP2K5; GIPR; FANCL; SDCCAG8; TNKS-MSRA; TNN13K; LRRN6C; NRXN3 FLJ35779; SLC39A8; TMEM160; CADM2; LRP1B; PRKD1; MTIF3; ZNF608; PTBP2; TUB; HMGA1; PPYR1
Associated with childhood obesity – novel loci	SH2B1; EDIL3; S1PR5; FOXP2; TBCA; ABCB5; ZPLD1; KIF2B; ARL15; EPHA6-UNQ6114
Associated with childhood and/or adult waist to hip ratio	LYPLAL1; C12orf51; LY86
Chromosome location and gene for phenotype gene relationships	**Gene or chromosome location**
Obesity, early onset	1p36.11 (NROB2); 2p23.3 (POMC)
Obesity, severe	3p25.2 (PPARG); 6q16.3 (SIM1); 11q13.4 (ULP3)
Obesity	1p35.2 (SDC3); 3p25.3 (GHRL); 4q31.1 (UCP1); 5q13.2 (CART); 5q32 (ADRB2; PPARGC1B); 6q23.2 (ENPP1); 8p11.23 (ADRB3); 13q14 (OLFM4); 16q22.1 (AGRP); 17q21 (HOXB5); 17q21.31 (PYY); 18q21.32 (MC4R)

Historically, three approaches to treat obesity have been tried with some level of success at least in the short term. These include lifestyle changes with diets, pharmacological agents and bariatric surgery procedures. Predisposing genetic factors for weight gain and development of obesity in humans also can impact on the response to intervention in terms of weight loss. For example, individuals with *MC4R* or *POMC* mutations appear to respond to a reduced caloric diet and exercise program but those with *MC4R* mutations fail to maintain weight lost after intervention [2]. Access to a multidisciplinary team may be helpful in achieving weigh loss including genetic evaluations and screening for obesity-related disorders or monogenic causes, dietary consultation and behavior/pharmaceutical therapy and, if indicated, bariatric surgery as a final option for exogenous obesity.

Progress in genetic evaluations and testing will help to identify DNA factors contributing to obesity specific for each individual at risk in an "obesogenic" environment which is common in our modern society including environmental chemicals and heavy metals [39]. Next generation DNA sequencing and established whole-genome approaches have the potential to generate a comprehensive genetic map of predisposing causative factors for obesity and a more detailed picture of the biological mechanisms involved in the development of childhood obesity and eating behavior.

GENE-DIET INTERACTION

Childhood overweight and obesity have reached epidemic proportions worldwide and research studies indicate that the cause of the childhood obesity epidemic which has been emerging over the past 30 years is complex and results from an interaction of susceptibility genes with an environment which is conducive for the development of obesity [40]. For much of this time, the primary causes of childhood obesity remained unknown but early studies suggested psychology was responsible for overconsumption of food but more recent studies using data from twins fed different diets and/or raised independently further confirms that genetics play a role [41]. However, it is unlikely that genetic mutations alone could account for the recent obesity epidemic in our society as the genetics would not have changed so rapidly but existing genetic factors could interact with the current environment with increased availability of calorie-dense food and a more sedentary lifestyle requiring fewer calories. The obesogenic environment also takes into consideration gene-diet and gene-physical activity of each at-risk individual [42].

A previously proposed group of genes have been suggested to play a prominent role in the onset of obesity, i.e., the "thirty genes", which may permit efficient conversion of calories into stored fat particularly during time when food supplies are plentiful [43]. It is thought that the stored fat would then be readily available as an energy source when food sources became scarce. Hence, when exposed to a high-fat diet and sedentary lifestyle as components of our current obesogenic environment then excessive fat would be stored which could serve as an energy source if a famine did occur in the future. The existence of the so called "thrifty genes" could then become selected for certain groups of people due to natural evolution including the Pima Indians of Arizona who appear to be at greater risk for excessive weight gain, obesity and associated type 2 diabetes mellitus [44].

A number of genes are thought to be associated with either weight gain or obesity with a few showing an interaction with diet and thus contribute to childhood obesity [45]. One of these potential genes that contributes to the common (non-dysmorphic) forms of obesity is the *FTO* gene and was the first gene characterized in playing this role [28,46]. The *FTO* gene is located on chromosome 16q12.2 and expressed in most tissues with the highest amounts found in the arcuate hypothalamus of the brain [28]. It appears to be regulated by the fasting and feeding cycles in humans including several single nucleotide polymorphisms (SNPs) associated with promoting weight gain such as the SNP variant (rs9939609) found to influence satiety, appetite control and maintaining energy balance in several studies [47]. Further studies with subcutaneous adipose tissue biopsies obtained from healthy subjects suggested that the FTO protein coded by the *FTO* gene had a role in regulating the hydrolysis of triacylglycerols or triglycerides within the adipocytes and fat metabolism [48]. Interestingly, individuals who possess specific *FTO* gene variants appear to have an increased preference for calorie-dense foods such as fat and exhibiting decreased satiety. These specific genetic factors are responsible for promoting weight gain including childhood obesity and continued investigation of gene-diet interactions will be important to identify the interaction of specific genetic variations and candidate genes.

EXAMPLES OF OBESITY-RELATED GENETIC DISORDERS

Prader-Willi syndrome (PWS) was first reported in 1956 and is a neurodevelopmental disorder due to errors in genomic imprinting with loss of paternally expressed genes from chromosome 15, usually from a de novo 15q11-q13 deletion [49-53].

PWS is characterized by a range of mild learning problems, characteristic behavior including self-injury, outbursts, obsessive-compulsions, temper tantrums and hyperphagia and particular clinical findings such as short stature, small hands and feet, hypogonadism, hypotonia and feeding difficulties during infancy. Obesity which can be life-threatening occurs in early childhood if not controlled [51-54]. PWS is found in about 1 in 10,000 to 30,000 individuals and affects about 400,000 people worldwide [50,55]. Although most cases are sporadic, PWS is considered one of the most common known genetic causes of marked obesity. It affects all races and ethnic groups [50,53,54].

Fragile X syndrome (FXS) is the most common cause of familial intellectual disability in humans due to a triplet repeat mutation found in the *FMR1* gene located at chromosome Xq27.3 and associated with obesity. It generally affects males. FXS was first reported in 1969 [56] and is found in about 1 in 4,000 males in the general population [57,58]. Prominent features besides intellectual disability include prominent large ears, a narrow head and flat mid-face and prognathism, joint laxity and macro-orchidism. Autism can also be a common finding [59]. In addition, a subset of males with this gene mutation also presents with features similarly seen in Prader-Willi syndrome including hypotonia, developmental delay, behavioral problems, excessive eating and marked obesity [60,61].

Alström syndrome (AS) is a separate obesity related disorder due to a single gene (*ALMS1*) defect located on chromosome 2p13 and occurs in about 1 in 1,000,000 individuals [62]. The condition is characterized by multi-organ involvement, progressive vision and hearing loss, obesity in childhood with insulin resistance and type 2 diabetes mellitus and high lipid levels, hypogonadism, short stature and cardiac, liver, lung and kidney problems complicated by fibrotic changes [63].

The protein encoded by the *ALMS1* gene is related to ciliary function as seen in another genetic obesity disorder, Bardet-Biedl syndrome [64]. The clinical and genetic findings seen in the three obesity-related genetic disorders are shown in Table 2.

Table 2. Clinical, Learning, Behavior and Genetic Findings seen in Prader-Willi Syndrome, the Prader-Willi Phenotype in Fragile X Syndrome and Alström Syndrome

	Facial Features	Physical Features	Learning/Behavior Features	Genetics
Prader-Willi Syndrome	Narrow forehead, almond shaped eyes, strabismus, short nose with thin upper lip, downturned corners of mouth, dry sticky saliva, enamel hypoplasia	Severe hypotonia, short stature, obesity, osteoporosis, small hands and feet, scoliosis, hypopigmentation, head tilt forward, hypogenitalism	Mild learning impairment, hyperphagia, skin and rectal picking, difficulty with transitions, stubbornness, temper tantrums, perseverative speech, autism, obsessive-compulsions, unusual skill with jigsaw puzzles, high pain tolerance	Paternally derived 15q11-q13 deletion (70% of cases), maternal disomy 15 (about 25% of cases), imprinting defects (5% of cases)
Prader-Willi Phenotype (in Fragile X Syndrome)	Round face, almond shaped eyes, prominent ears	Obesity, delayed puberty, small penis, hypotonia	Developmental delay, food seeding behavior and hyperphagia, difficulty with transitions, perseverative speech, hand flapping, poor eye contact, autism, obsessive-compulsions	FMR1 gene triplet repeat mutations (at chromosome Xq27.3)
Alström Syndrome	Round face, deep-set eyes, thickened skull, thick ears, frontal hair loss	Wide, flat feet with brachydactyly, scoliosis, dental anomalies, truncal obesity, short suture, hypogonadism, cardiomyopathy, vision (cone-rod dystrophy) and hearing loss, type 2 diabetes, progressive pulmonary, renal and hepatic problems with fibrosis	Developmental delay, balance disturbances and neurosensory deficits, depression, autism, obsessive-compulsions	ALMS1 gene mutations (at chromosome 2p13)

Prader-Willi Syndrome

Prader-Willi syndrome (PWS) occurs from paternal lack of expression of genes known to be imprinted in the 15q11-q13 region whereby the phenotype is modified depending on which parent contributes the genetic information to the offspring [52,65,66]. PWS is recognized as the most common known cause of morbid obesity in childhood [50]. Epigenetic changes controlling gene expression is reversible in gametogenesis without changing the DNA sequence usually through DNA methylation [67]. Imprinted genes impacted by the sex of the parent are mono-allelically expressed and errors in imprinting due to mutations or deletions can lead to different phenotypic outcomes or syndromes (i.e., PWS with loss of paternal expression of genes in the 15q11-q13 region and Angelman syndrome, an entirely different clinical disorder due to loss of maternal expression of genes in the same chromosome region) [68]. Errors in genomic imprinting were first reported in humans involving this chromosome region in PWS and Angelman syndrome and have led to the discovery of causation in other human disorders and diseases [69,70].

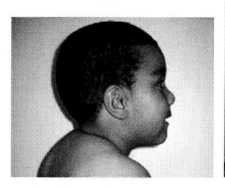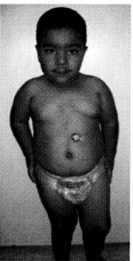

Figure 1. Frontal and profile views of a 4 year old male with Prader-Willi syndrome due to maternal disomy 15 and treated with growth hormone since early infancy. Note the facial appearance, gastrostomy and central obesity which are characteristic of children with this rare obesity-related genetic disorder.

Classical features of PWS include hypotonia and feeding difficulties with a poor suck during infancy, a particular facial appearance, developmental delay and hypogonadism with hypogenitalism in both males and females. Later, hyperphagia and onset of obesity occurs in early childhood along with short stature, small hands and feet due to growth hormone deficiency, mild learning deficits and behavioral problems (e.g., skin picking, obsessive compulsions, temper tantrums, stubbornness). The characteristic facial features include a small upturned nose, dolichocephaly with a narrow forehead and almond-shaped eyes, a thin upper lip, down-turned corners of the mouth and decreased sticky saliva. The skin, hair and eye color is usually lighter than seen in other family members which correlates with those having the 15q11-q13 deletion [50, 53, 54, 71] (Figure 1).

Clinical Stages and Natural History

Obesity is the most significant health problem in PWS but initially failure-to-thrive and feeding problems are seen. Historically, the clinical course for this disorder has been divided into two distinct stages characterized by failure-to-thrive in infancy during the first stage and later, hyperphagia and early childhood obesity (second stage). Recently, the natural history of PWS has been further divided into seven nutritional phases characterized by five main phases and two sub-phases: Phase 0 is seen in the fetus with decreased activity and often with breech presentation; Phase 1 in infancy with hypotonia and feeding problems; Phase 2 with weight gain without a significant change in appetite beginning at about 2 years of age and an increased interest in food at about 4 years of age; Phase 3 with hyperphagia, food seeking and lack of satiety with a median age of onset at about 8 years of age; and Phase 4 in some adults and characterized by a lessening of the insatiable appetite [72]. With an earlier diagnosis due to better recognition and improved genetic testing and use of growth hormone to treat the growth failure in children with PWS, changes are seen in the clinical course development. Additional studies are underway to further characterize the natural history.

Generally, the second stage in clinical course development in non-growth hormone treated PWS begins around 2 years of age [71]. This stage is characterized by continued developmental delay and onset of hyperphagia which leads to obesity if not controlled, but infants with PWS are often born in breech presentation with severe central hypotonia, temperature instability, a poor suck and hypogonadism/hypogenitalism. Due to developmental delay, they sit independently by 1 year of age, crawl at 16 months and walk at about 2 years and talk (10 words) at 39 months [50,71]. The clinical features seen in

PWS do show marked variability throughout the life span with the phenotype evolving from birth to adulthood. Because of generalized hypotonia and decreased muscle mass, respiratory distress, swallowing problems and possible asphyxia may occur during illnesses if present. Central adrenal insufficiency has also been reported in about 10% of infants with PWS and should be monitored [73].

PWS infants generally have a weak or absent cry with little spontaneous activity due to decreased muscle tone and strength, excessive sleepiness with diminished swallowing and sucking reflexes [52-54]. Often necessitated, gavage feedings and use of special nipples or gastrostomy tube placement are required to address the feeding problems and to supply adequate nutrition for growth and development in the PWS infant. Growth parameters should be assessed regularly (weekly) using standardized growth charts developed for infants with PWS [74] during the first 6 months of life and then monthly. Calories are adjusted accordingly, but fats should not be restricted even though the non-growth hormone treated infant with PWS usually requires less than the recommended allowance to avoid rapid weight gain due to decreased metabolism and caloric requirement. Vitamin and mineral intake (e.g., calcium) as well as caloric intake should be monitored closely by a dietition. With progression through the descriptive nutritional phases recorded in the non-growth hormone treated individuals with PWS and with increased interest in food along with decreased caloric requirement (about 60% of normal), obesity can develop rapidly in early childhood. Hyperphagia becomes a major behavioral problem in PWS but, to date, no known pharmacological agent has been effective. Developmental assessments and early stimulation programs along with occupational and physical therapy services are recommended [51,54].

Endocrine disturbances in the production of thyroid, growth and sex hormones and adrenal problems are usually recognized early. Myopia and impaired stereoscopic vision maybe diagnosed in early childhood. Hypopigmentation is more pronounced at this time and correlates with those having the parental 15q11-q13 deletion [75]. Academic achievement is usually impaired during the first 6 years of life with the majority of individuals functioning in the mild-to-moderate range with the average IQ of 65. There are reported differences in behavior, academic achievement, and cognition between those with different genetic subtypes [76]. Many children begin school in mainstream settings, but special education and support services are often required. Children with PWS have relatively strong reading, visual and long-term memory skills, but have weaker math, sequential processing, and short-term memory skills. Verbal skills may be relative strengths as well as an unusual skill of working with jigsaw puzzles [54,77].

During adolescence, hypogonadism and hypogenitalism becomes more pronounced in the vast majority of individuals with PWS due to hypothalamic hypogonadism leading to low testosterone and estrogen levels. Cryptorchidism is present in about 90% of males accompanied with a small penis and underdeveloped scrotum. Hypoplastic labia majora and minora and a small clitoris are seen in most PWS females. Puberty is absent or delayed in both males and females with PWS and infertility is nearly always present. Menarche in females with PWS may occur but delayed until 30 years of age. Little data are available about sexual activity in PWS, but an interest is shown by establishing relationships and demonstrating affection. In rare cases, pregnancies in females with PWS have been reported [54, 78].

Approximately 90% of non-growth hormone treated individuals with PWS will develop short stature by adulthood with the average adult male being 155 cm tall and the adult female at 147 cm [79]. Small hands and feet or acromicria are more pronounced during adolescence and adulthood accompanied by scoliosis and kyphosis which may require treatment (bracing or surgery). Without intervention, adolescents with PWS may weigh more than 300 pounds impacting on morbidity and mortality. Eating related fatalities do occur including choking on gorged food and gastric necrosis and rupture [80]. Therefore to avoid these complications, locking the refrigerator and food cabinets to prevent excessive eating are often undertaken with close supervision. Because of the abnormal eating behavior and complications related to obesity, adult independent living arrangements are prescribed. Therefore, weight and behavior problems need to be adequately addressed which are characteristic of PWS and requires involvement of not only the patient but family members and care providers. Although psychotropic agents can be helpful in controlling abnormal behavior seen in PWS, no specific medication has been consistently effective in controlling food-seeking behavior [51, 54, 81].

To address the multiple health related problem seen in PWS, management requires a multidisciplinary approach with goals to control weight gain and monitoring or treating associated comorbid conditions, controlling behavioral problems and for replacement of deficient growth and sex hormones. Rigorous control of the food environment and adequate regular exercise programs are essential strategies to manage the hyperphagia and obesity, complications of which represent the major causes of morbidity and mortality in PWS [51, 54].

Mild mental deficiency for the family background and other behavioral problems seen in PWS and often include obsessive- compulsions, sudden outbursts which may be triggered by withholding food, lying, stealing, tantrums, and self-injury beginning in childhood. Children with PWS are often affectionate but less agreeable and more rigid than other children. In addition, speech problems, food foraging, daytime sleepiness and decreased physical activity are commonly seen. Other features include increased pain threshold with skin and rectal picking, temperature instability, strabismus, hypopig-mentation (particularly in those with the 15q11-q13 deletion), scoliosis which can worsen with growth hormone therapy, sleep apnea, and oral pathology with dental problems [51, 53, 82]. Behavioral problems may begin by age 3 years of age, and later, poor peer relationships, immaturity, and inappropriate social behavior are often noted. The craniofacial findings seen in PWS such as dolichocephaly, a narrow minimal frontal diameter, strabismus, almond-shaped eyes, short upturned nose with a thin upper lip and downturned corners of the mouth and dry, sticky salvia with enamel hypoplasia are also more pronounced during this time in early childhood [50].

Genetics

Prader-Willi syndrome is due to errors in genomic imprinting with loss of parentally expressed genes from the 15q11-q13 region. Genomic imprinting is an epigenetic phenomenon with the phenotype dependent on the sex of the parent contributing the gene allele to the offspring. Epigenetic effects are heritable changes in gene expression which can be reversed and influenced by the environment such as nutrition (e.g., folate). The changes are not associated with DNA sequence alterations. The effects are reversible and occur during gametogenesis mediated by several molecular processes, including DNA methylation, histone modification and/or RNA silencing. Nearly all imprinted genes have a CpG-rich differentially methylated region or key regulatory areas which control gene activity, and when methylated, inactivates the expression of the gene. The epigenetic phenomenon evolved about 150 million years ago with about 1% of mammalian genes thought to be imprinted. Imprinted genes are known to affect viability, growth and development which impact on other obesity-related and overgrowth disorders such as Albright hereditary osteodystrophy and Beckwith-Weidemann syndrome [66,68].

Most of the genes or transcripts from the chromosome 15q11-q13 region are subject to genomic imprinting and disturbances lead to human disease such as PWS with loss of alleles only active on the paternal chromosome 15. These same alleles found on the maternal chromosome 15 are silenced by epigenetic factors (primarily through methylation). Conversely, loss of expression of one of the two preferentially maternally expressed genes in the 15q11-q13 region (i.e., the *UBE3A* gene) usually by the same chromosome 15 deletion but of maternal origin leads to Angelman syndrome (AS), the second genomic imprinting disorder identified in humans [70].

The chromosome 15q11-q13 region contains about 8 million DNA base pairs and dozens of genes/transcripts including a cluster of imprinted genes under the control of two imprinting controlling centers (one for PWS and one for AS) and a non-imprinted domain of genes which are expressed equally from either the maternal or paternal chromosome 15 [83]. Novel low copy DNA repeat sequences are located in this chromosome region at designated sites [52]. These areas contain the functional *HERC2* gene located distally at breakpoint BP3 and two HERC2 pseudogenes located at two proximal breakpoint sites (BP1 and BP2) in the 15q11-q13 region [84,85]. These chromosome 15 breakpoints contain similar DNA sequences, which contribute to non-homologous pairing and aberrant recombination or crossing-over events during meiosis. This mis-pairing leads to deletions in the offspring causing PWS when present on the father's chromosome 15 (or AS if present on the mother's chromosome 15).

About 70% of PWS individuals will show a typical *de novo* paternal deletion of the 15q11-q13 region consisting of two types, type I and type II [52,53,65]. The type I deletion is larger and involves chromosome breakpoints BP1 and BP3 while the type II deletion is smaller in size and involves breakpoints BP2 and BP3. Four genes (*TUBGCP5, CYFIP1, NIPA1, NIPA2*) are located between BP1 and BP2 (Figure 2). These four genes are not imprinted but have biallelic or normal expression from both the maternal and paternal chromosome 15s. Individuals with speech delay and autistic findings having recently been reported having deletions and/or duplications of only the four genes between BP1 and BP2. In about 5% of individuals with PWS, an unusual or atypical deletion can be seen which is greater or smaller in size than the typical type I or type II deletion [52,53,86].

The second most common genetic cause of PWS is maternal disomy 15 where both chromosome 15s come from the mother and found in about 25% of individuals with PWS [65]. There are three recognized forms of maternal disomy 15. These include maternal heterodisomy 15 with two different chromosome 15s from the mother due to errors in the first stage of meiosis (meiosis I) from non-disjunction and without cross-over events or shuffling of genes from the two maternal chromosome 15s. A second form is maternal isodisomy 15 with two identical chromosome 15s from the mother due to errors in the second division of meiosis (meiosis II) or the equational phase due to non-disjunction. The third form is segmental maternal isodisomy 15 with two partially different chromosome 15s received in the offspring from the mother due to errors in meiosis I from non-disjunction with cross-over events leading to segments of isodisomy or DNA sequence regions with identical gene alleles. An abnormal genetic result can occur if the mother is a carrier of an autosomal recessive gene mutation for a disorder on chromosome 15 and located in the isodisomic region. This leads to identical DNA sequences and the same gene alleles. The PWS child would then have a second genetic condition besides PWS [52].

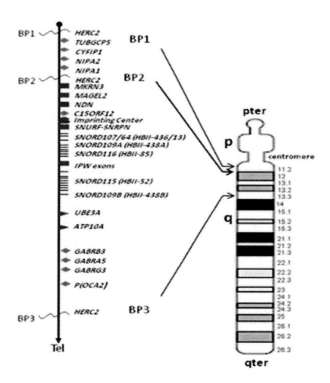

Figure 2. Chromosome 15 ideogram showing the location of genes in the 15q11-q13 region. BP1, BP2 and BP3 are the three common chromosome 15 breakpoints in the region at the site of breakage leading to the larger typical type I deletion between BP1 and BP3 and the smaller type II deletion between BP2 and BP3. The blue colored rectangle-shaped symbols represent paternally expressed genes (e.g., *MAGEL2*) which when disturbed leads to Prader-Willi syndrome. The red colored triangle-shaped symbols represent maternally expressed genes and the *UBA3E* gene when disturbed causes Angelman syndrome. The green colored diamond-shaped symbols represent genes (e.g., *CYFIP1*) expressed on both the maternal and paternal chromosome 15s.

Maternal disomy 15 is thought to arise from an error in gametogenesis in the female with the egg containing two chromosome 15s from the mother and if fertilized by a normal sperm with a single chromosome 15 then a trisomy 15 zygote results [87]. Trisomy 15 is lethal and a relatively common cause of spontaneous abortions. In an event of trisomy 15 rescue, the extra chromosome 15 is not passed in the next cell division in the developing embryo. Thus, a normal 46 chromosome number is now established in the embryo from an abnormal 47 chromosome count and leads to viability of the fetus. If the father's chromosome 15 is lost then the two remaining chromosome 15s from the mother will lead to maternal disomy 15 and the fetus is born with Prader-Willi syndrome due to his genetic subtype.

Another genetic phenomenon can occur in females with PWS due to maternal disomy 15 which involves the X chromosome. Females have two X chromosomes (one from the father and one from the mother) while males have only one X chromosome; however, the number of active X-linked genes remains constant in both sexes due to gene dosage compensation in females with or without PWS. Females generally inactivate one of their X chromosomes at random which then equals the number of X-linked genes found in the male. This process of X chromosome inactivation occurs very early in pregnancy. Occasionally, this process is not random and skewness occurs which can allow for expression of X-linked conditions in females. Hence, the trisomy 15 rescue event in the early pregnancy of a developing female with PWS and maternal disomy 15 may allow for a small number of cells to survive and to populate embryo development. These small number of cells rescued by the trisomy event may have the same X chromosome active leading to X chromosome inactivation skewness. This allows for the presence of an X-linked condition if the mother is a carrier of an X-linked gene and PWS due to maternal disomy 15 [88].

The third major category of genetic subtypes in PWS is an imprinting defect. These defects may be due to microdeletions of the imprinting center or due to epimutations through DNA methylation errors in gametogenesis. If the father carries an imprinting defect (microdeletion) that he inherits from his mother's chromosome 15, he is unaffected due to the presence of his father's normal chromosome 15. However, when he passes the imprinting defect in his chromosome 15 onto his offspring that offspring will then have PWS. The risk for him to pass the defect to his offspring would be 50% [52].

Limited information is available regarding genotype-phenotype correlations in PWS with those having the typical chromosome 15 deletion are hypopigmented and more homogeneous [50,75,89] while those with maternal disomy have fewer typical facial features and less likely to have skin picking, unusual skill with jigsaw puzzles, a high pain threshold or articulation problems. Based on clinical presentation, PWS individuals with maternal disomy are usually diagnosed later in life reflecting a milder phenotype. Those with the 15q11-q13 deletion have a greater number of compulsive symptoms than those with maternal disomy 15 and lower verbal IQ scores [90,91] but PWS children with the deletion possess relative strengths in visual-spatial tasks and object assembly [92].

Those subjects with PWS with the larger type I deletion are reported with more behavioral problems than those with the smaller type II deletion or maternal disomy 15, including skin picking, obsessive-compulsive traits and maladaptive behavior [91]. However, those individuals with PWS due to maternal disomy 15 show neuroanatomical differences in brain imaging with lower gray and white matter volume than those with the 15q11-q13 deletion. This could impact on speech, memory and concentration as the gray cerebral matter is related to general intelligence.

Molecular testing for PWS should begin with DNA methylation analysis of blood or other biological specimens. This testing is 99% accurate for the diagnosis of PWS [54] but does not distinguish among genetic subtypes (deletion, maternal disomy or imprinting defect). If the DNA methylation test is normal (not PWS), then other clinical disorders should be considered to account for the clinical presentation. A chromosome analysis with FISH to identify the 15q11-q13 deletion is often ordered to rule out a chromosome 15 translocation or to identify another rearrangement such as an inversion. DNA or chromosomal microarrays using both copy number or polymorphic probes are now used to identify the 15q11-q13 deletion and to identify the presence of maternal disomy 15 in selected individuals. Genotyping with polymorphic DNA markers from PWS family members (affected child, father and mother) can be helpful in identifying the imprinting defect in the presence of an abnormal (PWS) methylation pattern. The use of polymorphic DNA markers can distinguish if the PWS child has biparental (normal) inheritance of the chromosome 15 or if both chromosome 15s are from the mother.

Dozens of genes/transcripts are located in the 15q11-q13 region including four normally expressed genes (NIPA1, NIPA2, CYFIP1, GCP5); five protein coding genes that are imprinted and paternally expressed (*MKRN3, MAGEL2, NDN,* and the bicistronic *SNURF-SNRPN*), a cluster of five snoRNA genes (*SNORD109, SNORD64, SNORD109A, SNORD116* and *SNORD115*) and several antisense transcripts including for the *UBE3A* gene; two maternally expressed and imprinted genes (*UBE3A* and *ATP10A)* and three non-imprinted gamma aminobutyric acid (GABA) receptor subunit genes (*GABRB3, GABRA5, GABRG3*), *P* (pigment) and *HERC2* [52,53,65] (See Figure 2).

An important gene, the *SNRPN* (small nuclear ribonucleoprotein N) and a second protein coding sequence (*SNURF*, or *SNRPN* upstream reading frame) and copies of the C/D box small nucleolar RNAs (snoRNAs) or *SNORDs* are involved in RNA processing which is key in causing the PWS phenotype with brain development and function [93]. Necdin (*NDN*) is also paternally expressed and involved with axonal growth with over expression in the hypothalamus, thalamus and pons and implicated in neonatal lethality and respiratory problems in mice [94]. The *MAGEL2* gene is paternally expressed in the brain (hypothalamus) and may play a role in circadian rhythm, brain development and fertility in humans. The *MKRN3* gene encodes specific proteins (makorins) that are abundantly expressed in the brain [52,66].

Mutations of the *UBE3A* gene are known to cause Angelman syndrome while other genes are located in the distal area of the 15q11-q13 region including *GABRB3, GABRA5* and *GABRG3*. GABA is a major inhibitory neurotransmitter. Alterations in GABA function are associated with hunger, obsessive-compulsions and abnormal vision and memory. The *P* gene which is involved with pigment production is also located in this region and deleted in both PWS and AS individuals but it is not imprinted and expressed on both the mother's and father's chromosome 15. Therefore, several of the genes (imprinted or not imprinted) found in the 15q11-q13 region deleted in most individuals with PWS appear to contribute to the PWS phenotype as PWS is not due to a single gene [52] (See Figure 2).

Limited information is available regarding genotype-phenotype correlations in PWS and those having the typical chromosome 15 deletion with either the longer type I or smaller type II or maternal disomy 15 but a few differences have been reported. For example, those with the typical 15q11-q13 deletion present with hypopigmentation and more homogeneous clinical findings than seen in the other genetic subtypes including a more typical facial appearance, more self-injurious behavior (skin picking), higher pain threshold and greater jigsaw puzzle skills. There are two typical 15q11-q13 deletions seen in PWS subjects and those with the longer type I deletions have increased maladaptive and compulsive behaviors or poorer academic performance relative to the smaller type II deletions or maternal disomy 15. Those with type II deletions show better adaptive behavior and social skills relative to those with type I or maternal disomy 15. Those with maternal disomy 15 have higher verbal IQ scores, greater numeric calculation skills, superior visual memory, poorer object assembly and visual perceptual skills and increased psychosis relative to those PWS subjects with the typical 15q11-q13 deletion (either type I or type II) [91,95].

Molecular testing for PWS to confirm the diagnosis should begin with DNA methylation analysis which is 99% accurate for the diagnosis but it does not identify the genetic subtype. Fluorescence *in situ* hybridization (FISH) to identify the 15q11-q13 deletion and chromosome analysis can be used to rule out a chromosome 15 translocation or other rearrangement. Presently, DNA or chromosomal microarrays are commonly used with both CNV and SNP probes to identify the 15q11-q13 deletion and to identify the presence of the maternal disomy 15 status in selected individuals. Genotyping with polymorphic DNA markers from PWS family members (child and parents) are helpful in identifying the imprinting defect in the presence of a PWS methylation pattern and by having normal inheritance of the chromosome 15.

Fragile X Syndrome and Prader-Willi Phenotype

As obesity is a cardinal feature of Prader-Willi syndrome (PWS), it is also common in a subset of individuals with the fragile X syndrome (FXS). A recent survey of body mass index (BMI) data collected from 718 children with FXS showed a prevalence rate of obesity (31%) which was higher than that found in age matched control children (18%) [96]. FXS is considered the most common cause of familial intellectual disability and due to a CGG triplet repeat expansion greater than 200 in size in the 5' untranslated region of the fragile X mental retardation 1 (*FMR1*) gene [57,58]. This expanded mutation usually leads to methylation and little to no mRNA is transcribed; thus, a lack of production of the fragile X mental retardation protein (FMRP) encoded by the *FMR1* gene [57,58]. Lack of this protein is correlated with an increased childhood growth rate in FXS patients and supported by evidence from the FXS knockout mouse model showing enhanced growth rate for the mice and with obesity. Interestingly, about 10% of individuals with FXS will have severe obesity, hyperphagia, hypogonadism or delayed puberty as similarly seen in PWS. This subset of FXS patients, termed the Prader-Willi phenotype (PWP), do not have chromosome 15q11-q13 gene deletions or abnormalities [58].

The *FMR1* gene is located at the chromosome Xq27.3 band consisting of 17 coding exons that span 38kb in size [97]. FMRP is transported back and forth between the nucleus and the cytoplasm with binding and transportation of mRNAs in the neurons at the synapse level in the brain. FMRP stabilizes mRNA or can enhance degradation of mRNA. It appears to shape the pattern of mRNA regulation throughout human fetal development [98]. Interestingly, a lower expression of a gene located in the 15q11-q13 region involved with PWS which encodes the cytoplasmic FMR1– interacting protein 1 (*CYFIP1*) also works in concert with FMRP and is associated with PWP [61].

The classic features seen in FXS patients include an elongated face with a prominent forehead and ears, flat feet, hyperextensible joints and macroorchidism. Characteristic behavioral findings include anxiety, attention deficit hyperactivity disorder, autistic tendencies such as hyperarousal to sensory stimuli including food texture and often obsessive-compulsive disorder [99]. These obsessions when focused on food can lead to overeating, food seeking at night and obesity which can be severe and, thus, the PWP status. PWP individuals are described as having a lack of satiation leading to hyperphagia by 5 years of age and truncal obesity involving the torso and abdomen as similarly seen in PWS by 10 years of age. Other PWP features in common with PWS include a round face, hypotonia, short stature, delayed puberty and hypogenitalism with a ravenous appetite including the consumption of inedible food such as raw meat and lack of satiety requiring locking refrigerators [58].

Alström Syndrome

Clinical

Alström syndrome is another rare obesity-related disorder due to a single gene defect with an inheritance pattern of autosomal recessive. It has a prevalence of less than 1 per 1,000,000 [62]. Due to multi-organ involvement, individuals with Alström syndrome have a reduced life expectancy of less than 50 years. This obesity syndrome is caused by mutations in the *ALMS1* gene located on chromosome 2p13 with symptoms occurring during infancy. Affected individuals have visual impairment, cone-rod dystrophy and hearing loss, childhood truncal obesity, insulin resistance and type 2 diabetes mellitus, hypertriglyceridemia, short stature, dilated cardiomyopathy, and progressive pulmonary, hepatic, and renal dysfunction with developing fibrosis in multiple organs [63,100].

The protein coded for by the *ALMS1* gene when disturbed involves organs throughout the body but its normal function is unclear. A role in ciliary function, intracellular trafficking and adipocyte differentiation has been reported [64,101] as observed in a second obesity-related genetic disorder with similar findings, Bardet-Biedl syndrome. The diagnosis of Alström syndrome is usually made based on clinical features and confirmed by molecular genetic testing of disease causing mutations in the *ALMS1* gene.

Obesity is a consistent health issue observed in most children with Alström syndrome [100] with significant and rapid weight gain beginning in the first year of life and predominantly distributed in both subcutaneous and visceral compartments. Severe insulin resistance with high insulin levels and impaired glucose tolerance are often observed in very early childhood in this syndrome. It is frequently accompanied by acanthosis nigricans, a cutaneous marker of insulin resistance at an early age. The mean age of onset of diabetes mellitus is about 16 years [63]. Metformin has been helpful but insulin may also be required for treatment. Dyslipiedemia or high lipid levels are seen at an early age with hypertriglyceridemia being sufficiently severe to cause pancreatitis [102] and also an increased risk for cardiovascular disease [62].

Other complex health issues include cardiomyopathy and congestive heart failure (CHF) in about 70% of individuals with this syndrome. This accounts for major causes of morbidity and mortality. The onset of CHF can occur as early as infancy or may develop later in adolescents or adults leading to fibrosis and myocardial hypertrophy with dilation and restrictive impairment of both ventricles [62,103]. Hepatic changes are also seen including cirrhosis, steatosis and hepatosplenomegaly followed by gastrointestinal bleeding, inflammation and fibrosis. End-stage liver disease is the cause of death in about 10% of individuals with Alström syndrome [63]. Renal disease is characterized by progressive renal impairment and varying degrees of glomerular disease, albuminuria and interstitial fibrosis. End-stage renal disease can occur as early as the teenage years and is also a major cause of morbidity. Hypogonadism is seen in both males and females with Alstrom syndrome, particularly with low-normal levels of testosterone and elevated gonadotropins in males having small penile length and testicular atrophy. Secondary sex characteristics are generally normal in males but are delayed. Hypogonadism in females may not become evident until pubertal age but with delay in secondary sex characteristics and menarche. Infertility is a consistent finding in Alström syndrome. Several endocrine disturbances are known to occur in Alström syndrome as well, including decreased growth velocity with advancing age. Most adolescents and adults are reported with short stature. Insulin-like growth factors and growth hormone levels are low. Hypothyroidism has also been reported. Chronic respiratory tract infections are common beginning in early childhood with some becoming severe leading to chronic bronchitis, asthma and obstructive pulmonary disease. Pulmonary hypertension is common with severe interstitial obliterating fibrosis reported, consistent with the fibrotic changes occurring in other major organs [62].

Most individuals with Alström syndrome are reported with a normal intelligence, although mild to moderate delay in reaching major milestones are sometimes noted including speech. Major depression, obsessive-compulsions and psychotic disturbances may occur particularly during adulthood. Balance disturbances are common [104] but without ataxia or impaired coordination. Cerebellar anomalies have been reported [105]. A particular facial appearance is recognized in Alström syndrome including deep-set eyes with a round face, a thickened skull, thick appearing ears and thin hair with premature frontal hair loss. Flat feet, brachydactyly, scoliosis and kyphosis are frequently observed. Dental anomalies including mal-aligned, missing, discolored or extra teeth may be present. Nystagmus and extreme photophobia are often noted along with visual dysfunction due to cone dystrophy and subnormal rod activity. Bilateral cataracts and complete blindness usually occurs by the second decade of life with the majority of individuals having slow progressive bilateral sensorineural hearing loss usually during the first decade. The age of onset and severity of these findings are variable [62,106].

Genetics

The *ALMS1* gene contains 23 exons with several alternatively spliced transcripts (isoforms) reported with the longest transcript producing a 461 kDa protein size consisting of 4169 amino acids [101,107]. Alström syndrome is due to mutations of this protein coding gene and is inherited in an autosomal recessive pattern. As with other recessive disorders, heterozygous carriers of mutations are generally asymptomatic. A large tandem repeat domain is found in exon 8 which encodes 34 imperfect repeats of about 50 amino acids in size which constitutes about 40% of the protein [101].

A conserved motif at the end of the protein which has been conserved in evolution shares sequences similarly seen in centrosomal proteins. This supports a role for the Alström syndrome gene and protein in cilia function in development of early onset childhood obesity. Centrosomes are cell organelles involved with microtubules which orchestrate aspects of chromosome movement during cell division and for development of signaling pathways impacting on primary cilium. Interestingly, the expression of the *ALMS1* gene is found in most tissues affected in individuals with Alström syndrome including the organ of Corti with associated hearing loss, retinal photoreceptors impacting on vision and in the kidney and liver [62,107-109].

There are over 100 different mutations reported in the *ALMS1* gene found in individuals with Alström syndrome [62]. The majority are of the nonsense or frameshift (insertion or deletion) type and most often involve the coding regions of exons 8, 10 and 16. Population studies in this gene have suggested founder effects in certain ethnic backgrounds with lack of disease causing mutations in the 5' half of the coding region of *ALMS1* (including exons 1-7). These observations prompt speculation that mutations in this specific gene region are lethal to the developing embryo [110].

Over 200 unique single nucleotide polymorphisms (SNPs) have been identified in the *ALMS1* gene with a trend for higher SNP density found in the 3' and of the coding region of the *ALMS1* gene suggesting an evolutionary impact with strong positive selection [62]. The prevalence of specific haplogroups for this gene may have occurred by selection about 15,000 years ago in Eurasian populations. One of the SNPs (rs7598660) was found to be weakly associated with several insulin and glucose related traits and linked to higher insulin levels with an ancestral allele also in Eurasian populations [62,111]. The selective pressure acting on *ALMS1* is unclear but other regions of selection in the human genome have been associated with carbohydrate metabolism. A possible variation in the *ALMS1* gene could have contributed to insulin resistance carried on a selected genetic haplotype. Hence, severe insulin resistance and impaired glucose intolerance are common in early childhood in individuals with Alström syndrome.

Genetic association studies have examined whether phenotypic variation seen in individuals with Alström syndrome could be attributed to specific mutations within the *ALMS1* gene and a suggestive correlation was found for mutations in exon 8 and normal renal function. Common SNP variations in loci tightly linked to the *ALMS1* gene have also been found to be associated with kidney disease including the SNP (rs13538) for renal filtration rate and a second SNP (rs10206899) which lies in close proximity to the gene for serum creatinine levels [112]. Several mouse models that recapitulate the features seen in Alström syndrome are under investigation to further examine mechanisms that cause the pathologic findings seen in this rare obesity-related genetic disorder.

In summary, as common or exogenous obesity represents an interaction of complex multi-factorial agents including susceptibility genes with an obesogenic environment characterized by increased consumption of high caloric foods and a sedentary lifestyle, genetic mutations and variants are becoming more recognized as playing a role in response to our emerging environment. Research with known dietary components (high-fat food or high saturated-fat food) and population-based studies are needed to identify and develop targeted treatment protocols for personalized nutritional or pharmaceutical therapy for individuals at an increased risk for genetic factors and developing childhood obesity. In addition, the growing evidence learned about the role of genes from single gene obesity-related disorders such as Alström, Prader-Willi and fragile X syndromes and mutations or gene variants present in the general population need to be better characterized and information applied in the clinical setting beginning in early childhood to avoid obesity and its manifestations.

REFERENCES

[1]   Zhao J, Grant SF. Genetics of childhood obesity. *Journal of Obesity*. 2011:845-48.

[2]   Choquet H, Meyre D. Genetics of obesity: what have we learned? *Current Genomics*. 2011a 12(3):169-79.

[3]   Finucane MM, Stevens GA, Cowan MJ, Danaei G, Lin JK, Paciorek CJ, et al. National, regional, and global trends in body-mass index since 1980: systematic analysis of health examination surveys and epidemiological studies with 960 country-years and 9.1 million participants. *Lancet.* 2011 377(9765):557-67.

[4]   de Onis M, Blossner M, Borghi E. Global prevalence and trends of overweight and obesity among preschool children. *American Journal of Clinical Nutrition*. 2010 92(5):1257-64.

[5]   Manco M, Dallapiccola B. Genetics of pediatric obesity. *Pediatrics.* 2012 130(1):123-33.

[6]   Farooqi S. Insights from the genetics of severe childhood obesity. *Hormone Research*. 2007;68 Suppl 5:5-7.

[7]   Bouchard C, Perusse L. Current status of the human obesity gene map. *Obesity Research*. 1996 4(1):81-90.

[8]   Rankinen T, Zuberi A, Chagnon YC, Weisnagel SJ, Argyropoulos G, Walts B, et al. The human obesity gene map: the 2005 update. *Obesity.* 2006 14:529-644.

[9]   Dasouki MJ, Youngs EL, Hovanes K. Structural chromosome abnormalities associated with obesity: report of four new subjects and review of literature. *Current Genomics*. 2011 12(3):190-203.

[10] Bochukova EG, Huang N, Keogh J, Henning E, Purmann C, Blaszcyk K, et al. Large, rare chromosomal deletions assoicaited with severe early-onset obesity. *Nature*. 2010 463:666-70.

[11] Bachmann-Gagescu R, Mefford HC, Cowan C, Glew GM, Hing AV, Wallace S, et al. Recurrent 200-kb deletions of 16p11.2 that include the SH2B1 gene are associated with developmental delay and obesity. *Genetics in Medicine*. 2010 12(10):641-47.

[12] Bachmann-Gagescu R, Phelps IG, Stearns G, Link BA, Brockerhoff SE, Moens CB, et al. The ciliopathy gene cc2d2a controls zebrafish photoreceptor outer segment development through a role in Rab8-dependent vesicle trafficking. *Human Molecular Genetics*. 2011 20(20):4041-55.

[13] van Vliet-Ostaptchouk JV, Hofker MH, van der Schouw YT, Wijmenga C, Onland-Moret NC. Genetic variation in the hypothalamic pathways and its role on obesity. *Obesity Reviews*. 2009 10(6):593-609.

[14] Cecil J, Dalton M, Finlayson G, Blundell J, Hetherington M, Palmer C. Obesity and eating behaviour in children and adolescents: contribution of common gene polymorphisms. *International Review of Psychiatry*. 2012 24(3):200-10.

[15] Choquet H, Meyre D. Molecular basis of obesity: current status and future prospects. *Current Genomics*. 2011b 12(3):154-68.

[16] Feinleib M, Garrison RJ, Fabsitz R, Christian JC, Hrubec Z, Borhani NO, et al. The NHLBI twin study of cardiovascular disease risk factors: methodology and summary of results. *American Journal of Epidemiology*. 1977 106(4):284-85.

[17] Beyerlein A, von Kries R, Ness AR, Ong KK. Genetic markers of obesity risk: stronger associations with body composition in overweight compared to normal-weight children. *PLoS One*. 2011 6(4):e19057.

[18] Stunkard AJ, Foch TT, Hrubec Z. A twin study of human obesity. *Journal of the American Medical Association*. 1986 256(1):51-4.

[19] Stunkard AJ, Sorensen TI, Hanis C, Teasdale TW, Chakraborty R, Schull WJ, et al. An adoption study of human obesity. *New England Journal of Medicine*. 1986 314(4):193-98.

[20] Stunkard AJ, Harris JR, Pedersen NL, McClearn GE. The body-mass index of twins who have been reared apart. *New England Journal of Medicine*. 1990 322(21):1483-87.

[21] Silventoinen K, Rokholm B, Kaprio J, Sorensen TI. The genetic and environmental influences on childhood obesity: a systematic review of

twin and adoption studies. *International Journal of Obesity.* 2010 34(1):29-40.

[22] Clement K, Vaisse C, Lahlou N, Cabrol S, Pelloux V, Cassuto D, et al. A mutation in the human leptin receptor gene causes obesity and pituitary dysfunction. *Nature.* 1998 392(6674):398-401.

[23] Krude H, Biebermann H, Luck W, Horn R, Brabant G, Gruters A. Severe early-onset obesity, adrenal insufficiency and red hair pigmentation caused by POMC mutations in humans. *Nature Genetics.* 1998 19(2):155-57.

[24] Montague CT, Farooqi IS, Whitehead JP, Soos MA, Rau H, Wareham NJ, et al. Congenital leptin deficiency is associated with severe early-onset obesity in humans. *Nature.* 1997 387(6636):903-08.

[25] Hinney A, Bettecken T, Tarnow P, Brumm H, Reichwald K, Lichtner P, et al. Prevalence, spectrum, and functional characterization of melanocortin-4 receptor gene mutations in a representative population-based sample and obese adults from Germany. *Journal of Clinical Endocrinology and Metabolism.* 2006 91(5):1761-69.

[26] Farooqi S, O'Rahilly S. Genetics of obesity in humans. *Endocrine Reviews.* 2006 27(7):710-18.

[27] Dina C, Meyre D, Gallina S, Durand E, Korner A, Jacobson P, et al. Variation in FTO contributes to childhood obesity and severe adult obesity. *Nature Genetics.* 2007 39(6):724-26.

[28] Frayling TM, Timpson NJ, Weedon MN, Zeggini E, Freathy RM, Lindgren CM, et al. A common variant in the FTO gene is associated with body mass index and predisposes to childhood and adult obesity. *Science.* 2007 316(5826):889-94.

[29] Scherag A, Dina C, Hinney A, Vatin V, Scherag S, Vogel CI, et al. Two new Loci for body-weight regulation identified in a joint analysis of genome-wide association studies for early-onset extreme obesity in French and German study groups. *PLoS Genetics.* 2010 6(4):e1000916.

[30] Heard-Costa NL, Zillikens MC, Monda KL, Johansson A, Harris TB, Fu M, et al. NRXN3 is a novel locus for waist circumference: a genome-wide association study from the CHARGE Consortium. *PLoS Genetics.* 2009 5(6):e1000539.

[31] Chambers JC, Elliott P, Zabaneh D, Zhang W, Li Y, Froguel P, et al. Common genetic variation near MC4R is associated with waist circumference and insulin resistance. *Nature Genetics.* 2008 40(6): 716-18.

[32] Meyre D, Delplanque J, Chevre JC, Lecoeur C, Lobbens S, Gallina S, et al. Genome-wide association study for early-onset and morbid adult obesity identifies three new risk loci in European populations. *Nature Genetics*. 2009 41(2):157-59.

[33] Thorleifsson G, Walters GB, Gudbjartsson DF, Steinthorsdottir V, Sulem P, Helgadottir A, et al. Genome-wide association yields new sequence variants at seven loci that associate with measures of obesity. *Nature Genetics*. 2009 41(1):18-24.

[34] Speliotes EK, Willer CJ, Berndt SI, Monda KL, Thorleifsson G, Jackson AU, et al. Association analyses of 249,796 individuals reveal 18 new loci associated with body mass index. *Nature Genetics*. 2010 42(11):937-48.

[35] Wang J, Mei H, Chen W, Jiang Y, Sun W, Li F, et al. Study of eight GWAS-identified common variants for association with obesity-related indices in Chinese children at puberty. *International Journal of Obesity*. 2012 36(4):542-47.

[36] Heid IM, Jackson AU, Randall JC, Winkler TW, Qi L, Steinthorsdottir V, et al. Meta-analysis identifies 13 new loci associated with waist-hip ratio and reveals sexual dimorphism in the genetic basis of fat distribution. *Nature Genetics*. 2010 42(11):949-60.

[37] Bradfield JP, Taal HR, Timpson NJ, Scherag A, Lecoeur C, Warrington NM, et al. A genome-wide association meta-analysis identifies new childhood obesity loci. *Nature Genetics*. 2012 44(5):526-31.

[38] Loos RJ, Rankinen T, Rice T, Rao DC, Leon AS, Skinner JS, et al. Two ethnic-specific polymorphisms in the human Agouti-related protein gene are associated with macronutrient intake. *American Journal of Clinical Nutrition*. 2005 82(5):1097-101.

[39] La Merrill M, Birnbaum LS. Childhood obesity and environmental chemicals. *Mount Sinai Journal of Medicine*. 2011 78(1):22-48.

[40] Ogden CL, Carroll MD, Curtin LR, Lamb MM, Flegal KM. Prevalence of high body mass index in US children and adolescents, 2007-2008. *Journal of the American Medical Association*. 2010 303(3):242-9.

[41] Bruch H. Psychological aspects of overeating and obesity. *Psychosomatics*. 1964 5:269-74.

[42] Garver WS. Gene-diet interactions in childhood obesity. *Current Genomics*. 2011 12(3):180-89.

[43] Neel JV. Diabetes mellitus: a "thrifty" genotype rendered detrimental by "progress"? *American Journal of Human Genetics*. 1962 14:353-62.

[44] Knowler WC, Pettitt DJ, Bennett PH, Williams RC. Diabetes mellitus in the Pima Indians: genetic and evolutionary considerations. *American Journal of Physical Anthropology*. 1983 62(1):107-14.

[45] Papoutsakis C, Dedoussis GV. Gene-diet interactions in childhood obesity: paucity of evidence as the epidemic of childhood obesity continues to rise. *Personalized Medicine*. 2007 4:133-46.

[46] Loos RJ, Bouchard C. FTO: the first gene contributing to common forms of human obesity. *Obesity Reviews* 2008 9(3):246-50.

[47] Bruning JC, Gautam D, Burks DJ, Gillette J, Schubert M, Orban PC, et al. Role of brain insulin receptor in control of body weight and reproduction. *Science*. 2000 289(5487):2122-25.

[48] Wahlen K, Sjolin E, Hoffstedt J. The common rs9939609 gene variant of the fat mass- and obesity-associated gene FTO is related to fat cell lipolysis. *Journal of Lipid Research*. 2008 49(3):607-11.

[49] Prader A, Labhart A, Willi H. Ein sydnrom von adipositas, kleinwuchs, kryptorchismus und oligophrenie nach myatonieartigem zustand im neugeborenenalter. *Schweizerische Medizinishce Wochenschrift*. 1956 6(3):1260-61

[50] Butler MG. Prader-Willi syndrome: current understanding of cause and diagnosis. *American Journal of Medical Genetics*. 1990 35(3):319-32.

[51] Goldstone AP, Holland AJ, Hauffa BP, Hokken-Koelega AC, Tauber M, speakers contributors at the Second Expert Meeting of the Comprehensive Care of Patients with PWS. Recommendations for the diagnosis and management of Prader-Willi syndrome. *Journal of Clinical Endocrinology and Metabolism*. 2008 93(11):4183-97.

[52] Butler MG. Prader-Willi syndrome: obesity due to genomic imprinting. *Current Genomics*. 2011 12(3):204-15.

[53] Cassidy SB, Schwartz S, Miller JL, Driscoll DJ. Prader-Willi syndrome. *Genetics in Medicine*. 2012 14(1):10-26.

[54] Butler MG, Lee PDK, Whitman BY. *Management of Prader-Willi Syndrome. 3rd Edition*. New York: Springer; 2006

[55] Whittington J, Holland A, Webb T, Butler J, Clarke D, Boer H. Cognitive abilities and genotype in a population-based sample of people with Prader-Willi syndrome. *Journal of Intellectual Disability Research*. 2004 48(Pt 2):172-87.

[56] Lubs HA. A marker X chromosome. *American Journal of Human Genetics*. 1969 21(3):231-44.

[57] Hagerman R, Hoem G, Hagerman P. Fragile X and autism: intertwined at the molecular level leading to targeted treatments. *Molecular Autism.* 2010 1(1):12.

[58] McLennan Y, Polussa J, Tassone F, Hagerman R. Fragile X syndrome. *Current Genomics.* 2011 12(3):216-24.

[59] Hagerman RJ, Hagerman PJ. *Fragile X Syndrome: Diagonsis, Treatment, and Research. 3rd Edition.* Baltimore: The Johns Hopkins University Press; 2002.

[60] de Vries BB, Fryns JP, Butler MG, Canziani F, Wesby-van Swaay E, van Hemel JO, et al. Clinical and molecular studies in fragile X patients with a Prader-Willi-like phenotype. *Journal of Medical Genetics.* 1993 30(9):761-66.

[61] Nowicki ST, Tassone F, Ono MY, Ferranti J, Croquette MF, Goodlin-Jones B, et al. The Prader-Willi phenotype of fragile X syndrome. *Journal of Developmental and Behavioral Pediatrics.* 2007 28(2):133-38.

[62] Marshall JD, Bronson RT, Collin GB, Nordstrom AD, Maffei P, Paisey RB, et al. New Alström syndrome phenotypes based on the evaluation of 182 cases. *Archives of Internal Medicine.* 2005 165(6):675-83.

[63] Marshall JD, Beck S, Maffei P, Naggert JK. Alström syndrome. *European Journal of Human Genetics.* 2007 15(12):1193-202.

[64] Collin GB, Cyr E, Bronson R, Marshall JD, Gifford EJ, Hicks W, et al. Alms1-disrupted mice recapitulate human Alström syndrome. *Human Molecular Genetics.* 2005 14(16):2323-33.

[65] Bittel DC, Butler MG. Prader-Willi syndrome: clinical genetics, cytogenetics and molecular biology. *Expert Reviews in Molecular Medicine.* 2005 7(14):1-20.

[66] Hanel ML, Wevrick R. The role of genomic imprinting in human developmental disorders: lessons from Prader-Willi syndrome. *Clinical Genetics.* 2001 59(3):156-64.

[67] Buiting K, Gross S, Lich C, Gillessen-Kaesbach G, el-Maarri O, Horsthemke B. Epimutations in Prader-Willi and Angelman syndromes: a molecular study of 136 patients with an imprinting defect. *American Journal of Human Genetics.* 2003 72(3):571-77.

[68] Butler MG. Genomic imprinting disorders in humans: a mini-review. *Journal Assisted Reproductive Genetics.* 2009 26(9-10):477-86

[69] Nicholls RD, Knoll JH, Butler MG, Karam S, Lalande M. Genetic imprinting suggested by maternal heterodisomy in nondeletion Prader-Willi syndrome. *Nature.* 1989 342(6247):281-85.

[70] Williams CA, Driscoll DJ, Dagli AI. Clinical and genetic aspects of Angelman syndrome. *Genetics in Medicine* 2010 12(7):385-95.

[71] Butler MG, Meaney FJ, Palmer CG. Clinical and cytogenetic survey of 39 individuals with Prader-Labhart-Willi syndrome. *American Journal of Medical Genetics.* 1986 23(3):793-809.

[72] Miller JL, Lynn CH, Driscoll DC, Goldstone AP, Gold JA, Kimonis V, et al. Nutritional phases in Prader-Willi syndrome. *American Journal of Medical Genetics Part A.* 2011 155A(5):1040-49.

[73] de Lind van Wijngaarden RF, Joosten KF, van den Berg S, Otten BJ, de Jong FH, Sweep CG, et al. The relationship between central adrenal insufficiency and sleep-related breathing disorders in children with Prader-Willi syndrome. *Journal of Clinical Endocrinology and Metabolism.* 2009 94(7):2387-93.

[74] Butler MG, Sturich J, Lee J, Myers SE, Whitman BY, Gold JA, et al. Growth standards of infants with Prader-Willi syndrome. *Pediatrics.* 2011 127(4):687-95.

[75] Butler MG. Hypopigmentation: a common feature of Prader-Labhart-Willi syndrome. *American Journal of Human Genetics.* 1989 45(1): 140-46.

[76] Roof E, Stone W, MacLean W, Feurer ID, Thompson T, Butler MG. Intellectual characteristics of Prader-Willi syndrome: comparison of genetic subtypes. *Journal of Intellectual Disability Research.* 2000 44 (Pt 1):25-30.

[77] Dykens EM. Are jigsaw puzzle skills 'spared' in persons with Prader-Willi syndrome? *Journal of Child Psychology and Psychiatry, and Allied Disciplines.* 2002 43(3):343-52.

[78] Greenswag LR. Adults with Prader-Willi syndrome: a survey of 232 cases. *Developmental Medicine and Child Neurology.* 1987 29(2): 145-52.

[79] Butler MG, Meaney FJ. Standards for selected anthropometric measurements in Prader-Willi syndrome. *Pediatrics.* 1991 88(4):853-60.

[80] Stevenson DA, Heinemann J, Angulo M, Butler MG, Loker J, Rupe N, et al. Gastric rupture and necrosis in Prader-Willi syndrome. *Journal of Pediatric Gastroenterology and Nutrition.* 2007 45(2):272-74.

[81] McCandless SE, Committee on G. Clinical report-health supervision for children with Prader-Willi syndrome. *Pediatrics.* 2011 127(1):195-204.

[82] Hall BD, Smith DW. Prader-Willi syndrome. A resume of 32 cases including an instance of affected first cousins, one of whom is of normal stature and intelligence. *Journal of Pediatrics.* 1972 81(2):286-93.

[83] Butler MG, Fischer W, Kibiryeva N, Bittel DC. Array comparative
      genomic hybridization (aCGH) analysis in Prader-Willi syndrome.
      American Journal of Medical Genetics Part A. 2008 146(7):854-60.
[84] Nicholls RD, Knepper JL. Genome organization, function, and
      imprinting in Prader-Willi and Angelman syndromes. *Annual Review of
      Genomics and Human Genetics.* 2001 2:153-75.
[85] Chai JH, Locke DP, Greally JM, Knoll JH, Ohta T, Dunai J, et al.
      Identification of four highly conserved genes between breakpoint
      hotspots BP1 and BP2 of the Prader-Willi/Angelman syndromes deletion
      region that have undergone evolutionary transposition mediated by
      flanking duplicons. *American Journal of Human Genetics.* 2003
      73(4):898-925.
[86] Sahoo T, del Gaudio D, German JR, Shinawi M, Peters SU, Person RE,
      et al. Prader-Willi phenotype caused by paternal deficiency for the HBII-
      85 C/D box small nucleolar RNA cluster. *Nature Genetics.* 2008
      40(6):719-21.
[87] Cassidy SB, Lai LW, Erickson RP, Magnuson L, Thomas E, Gendron R,
      et al. Trisomy 15 with loss of the paternal 15 as a cause of Prader-Willi
      syndrome due to maternal disomy. *American Journal of Human
      Genetics.* 1992 51(4):701-8.
[88] Butler MG, Theodoro MF, Bittel DC, Kuipers PJ, Driscoll DJ,
      Talebizadeh Z. X-chromosome inactivation patterns in females with
      Prader-Willi syndrome. *American Journal of Medical Genetics Part A.*
      2007 143(5):469-75.
[89] Cassidy SB. Prader-Willi syndrome. *Current Problems in Pediatrics.*
      1984 14(1):1-55.
[90] Dykens EM, Leckman JF, Cassidy SB. Obsessions and compulsions in
      Prader-Willi syndrome. *Journal of Child Psychology and Psychiatry,
      and Allied Disciplines.* 1996 37(8):995-1002.
[91] Butler MG, Bittel DC, Kibiryeva N, Talebizadeh Z, Thompson T.
      Behavioral differences among subjects with Prader-Willi syndrome and
      type I or type II deletion and maternal disomy. *Pediatrics.* 2004 113(3 Pt
      1):565-73.
[92] Dykens EM. Are jigsaw puzzle skills 'spared' in persons with Prader-
      Willi syndrome? *Journal of Child Psychology and Psychiatry, and
      Allied Disciplines.* 2002 43(3):343-52.
[93] Kishore S, Stamm S. The snoRNA HBII-52 regulates alternative
      splicing of the serotonin receptor 2C. *Science.* 2006 311(5758):230-2.

[94] Miller NL, Wevrick R, Mellon PL. Necdin, a Prader-Willi syndrome candidate gene, regulates gonadotropin-releasing hormone neurons during development. *Human Molecular Genetics.* 2009 18(2):248-60.

[95] Zarcone J, Napolitano D, Peterson C, Breidbord J, Ferraioli S, Caruso-Anderson M, et al. The relationship between compulsive behaviour and academic achievement across the three genetic subtypes of Prader-Willi syndrome. *Journal of Intellectual Disability Research.* 2007 51(Pt. 6):478-87.

[96] Raspa M, Bailey DB, Bishop E, Holiday D, Olmsted M. Obesity, food selectivity, and physical activity in individuals with fragile X syndrome. *American Journal on Intellectual and Developmental Disabilities.* 2010 115(6):482-95.

[97] Bassell GJ, Warren ST. Fragile X syndrome: loss of local mRNA regulation alters synaptic development and function. *Neuron.* 2008 60(2):201-14.

[98] De Rubeis S, Bagni C. Fragile X mental retardation protein control of neuronal mRNA metabolism: Insights into mRNA stability. *Molecular and Cellular Neurosciences.* 2010 43(1):43-50.

[99] Cordeiro L, Ballinger E, Hagerman R, Hessl D. Clinical assessment of DSM-IV anxiety disorders in fragile X syndrome: prevalence and characterization. *Journal of Neurodevelopmental Disorders.* 2011 3(1):57-67.

[100] Marshall JD, Maffei P, Collin GB, Naggert JK. Alström syndrome: genetics and clinical overview. *Current Genomics.* 2011 12(3):225-35.

[101] Hearn T, Renforth GL, Spalluto C, Hanley NA, Piper K, Brickwood S, et al. Mutation of ALMS1, a large gene with a tandem repeat encoding 47 amino acids, causes Alström syndrome. *Nature Genetics.* 2002 31(1):79-83.

[102] Paisey RB, Carey CM, Bower L, Marshall J, Taylor P, Maffei P, et al. Hypertriglyceridaemia in Alström's syndrome: causes and associations in 37 cases. *Clinical Endocrinology.* 2004 60(2):228-31.

[103] Loudon MA, Bellenger NG, Carey CM, Paisey RB. Cardiac magnetic resonance imaging in Alström syndrome. *Orphanet Journal of Rare Diseases.* 2009 4:14.

[104] Möller C. *Vestibular Testing in Children.* In: Pediatric Audiological Medicine. New Jersey: Wiley-Blackwell, 2009.

[105] Yilmaz C, Caksen H, Yilmaz N, Guven AS, Arslan D, Cesure Y. Alström syndrome assoiciated with cerebral involvement: an unusual presentiaon. *European Journal of Medical Genetics.* 2006 3:32-34.

[106] Koray F, Dorter C, Benderli Y, Satman I, Yilmaz T, Dinccag N, et al. Alström syndrome: a case report. *Journal of Oral Science.* 2001 43(3):221-24.

[107] Collin GB, Marshall JD, Ikeda A, So WV, Russell-Eggitt I, Maffei P, et al. Mutations in ALMS1 cause obesity, type 2 diabetes and neurosensory degeneration in Alström syndrome. *Nature Genetics.* 2002 31(1):74-8.

[108] Hearn T, Spalluto C, Phillips VJ, Renforth GL, Copin N, Hanley NA, et al. Subcellular localization of ALMS1 supports involvement of centrosome and basal body dysfunction in the pathogenesis of obesity, insulin resistance, and type 2 diabetes. *Diabetes.* 2005 54(5):1581-87.

[109] Jagger D, Collin G, Kelly J, Towers E, Nevill G, Longo-Guess C, et al. Alström Syndrome protein ALMS1 localizes to basal bodies of cochlear hair cells and regulates cilium-dependent planar cell polarity. *Human Molecular Genetics.* 2011 20(3):466-81.

[110] Joy T, Cao H, Black G, Malik R, Charlton-Menys V, Hegele RA, et al. Alström syndrome (OMIM 203800): a case report and literature review. *Orphan Journal of Rare Diseases.* 2002 1:49.

[111] Scheinfeldt LB, Biswas S, Madeoy J, Connelly CF, Schadt EE, Akey JM. Population genomic analysis of ALMS1 in humans reveals a surprisingly complex evolutionary history. *Molecular Biology and Evolution.* 2009 26(6):1357-67.

[112] International HapMap C, Frazer KA, Ballinger DG, Cox DR, Hinds DA, Stuve LL, et al. A second generation human haplotype map of over 3.1 million SNPs. *Nature.* 2007 449(7164):851-6.

In: Childhood Obesity   ISBN: 978-1-62618-874-7
Editor: Callum G. Jackson   © 2013 Nova Science Publishers, Inc.

Chapter 2

CARDIOMETABOLIC IMPACT OF CHILDHOOD OBESITY AND THE POTENTIAL ROLE OF EXERCISE

Monica T. Marin[1], Kyle L. Sunderland[2], Paul Dasari[1] and Kevin R. Short[1]*

[1]Oklahoma University Health Sciences Center, Oklahoma City Oklahoma
[2]Health and Exercise Science Department, University of Oklahoma, US

ABSTRACT

Obesity in children is a significant public health problem in the United States as the number of adolescents who are overweight has tripled in the last 30 years so that 17% (or 12.5 million) of children and adolescents aged 2—19 years are now classified as obese based on body mass index (BMI). Excess weight in adolescence frequently persists into young adulthood, and has a strong adverse cardiometabolic impact. Additionally, available data suggest that children may be living increasingly sedentary lifestyles, which may exacerbate the effects of obesity on health and function, both now and in the future. Therefore there is currently a need to understand the causes and consequences of childhood obesity and to develop effective intervention approaches to

* Corresponding Author: Kevin R. Short, PhD; Section of Pediatric Diabetes/Endocrinology; 1200 Children's Ave, Suite 4500; Oklahoma City, Oklahoma 73104; Phone: 405-271-8001 x 43094; Email: kevin-short@ouhsc.edu.

prevent its development and/or the pathological effects of obesity. The purpose of this review is to provide an integrated examination of how obesity affects the risk for cardiovascular and metabolic (diabetes and bone) diseases, with emphasis on the role of physical exercise as a prevention and treatment strategy. For example, atherosclerosis starts in childhood and obesity appears to accelerate the development of atherosclerotic lesions. It has also been shown that childhood obesity clusters with components of the metabolic syndrome, such as high concentration of low-density lipoprotein (LDL), low concentration of high-density lipoprotein (HDL), insulin resistance and hypertension. Obesity is also a major risk factor for pre-diabetes and type 2 diabetes (T2DM). In obese people, fasting and postprandial plasma glucose concentration are the best clinical predictors for the progression from insulin resistance to T2DM The glycemic control also determines the future risk of micro and macro vascular complications, which demonstrates the inter-connection between metabolic and cardiovascular systems. Understanding how obesity affects bone health in children has become increasingly important. Many of the available studies that have assessed the effect of childhood obesity on bone accrual have resulted in conflicting results. However, recent evidence has shown that bone is a metabolically active tissue that responds to hormones like insulin, and produces proteins that affect pancreatic and adipose tissues, and that these communication processes are disrupted in the presence of obesity. Thus, obesity has integrated effects on multiple organs and tissues. Since physical exercise promotes bone loading, stimulates better glycemic control, and has protective effects on lipid profile and the cardiovascular system, an important focus of our research and this review is on the potential benefits of exercise for improving the health of obese children.

INTRODUCTION

Childhood obesity has more than tripled in the last 30 years [90] so that approximately 17% of children and adolescents aged 2-19 years in United States are obese and nearly a third are overweight or obese. Obesity in childhood often persists into young adulthood [108]. Obesity contributes to the growing prevalence of diabetes (~9-13% of Americans), pre-diabetes (16% of adolescents and 30% of US adults) and metabolic syndrome (25-50% of overweight adolescents) [24, 68, 73]. This high rate of pre-diabetes in adolescents is alarming because of the association with dyslipidemia and hypertension, which portends an increased future risk of metabolic and vascular disease when left untreated. Equally alarming are reports that American teenagers spend 55% of waking hours in sedentary activities and perform only half of the recommended volume of moderate-to-vigorous activity [34, 75, 86]. Sedentary lifestyle is an established risk factor for all-cause mortality in adults [75]; therefore, it is critical to establish healthier behavior patterns during youth since obesity and low fitness are likely to carry forward into adulthood [35, 85, 109]. The purpose of this review is to provide an integrated examination of how obesity affects the risk for cardiovascular and metabolic (diabetes and bone) diseases, with emphasis on the role of physical exercise as a prevention and treatment strategy.

OBESITY AND CARDIOVASCULAR RISK

Adult obesity predicts cardiovascular disease (*e.g.*, myocardial infarction, stroke, cardiovascular deaths) [125]. Cardiovascular disease (CVD) is the leading cause of death and morbidity in the United States [89]. In adults, detectable abnormalities in vascular function (i.e., arterial stiffness and reduced endothelium-dependent vasodilation) typically precede the development of vascular anatomical pathology such as vascular lesions and increased carotid intimal-media thickness [43, 47, 53, 65].

Most of the clinical burden of CVD occurs in adulthood, but some of these risk factors may be present at a young age. In children, overt vascular anatomical changes are less likely to be present compared to adults [103]. However, obese children have some of the same pro-atherogenic changes linked to adult vascular disease, including insulin resistance, hyperlipidemia, hepatic steatosis, and elevated levels of vascular inflammatory and fibrinolytic markers [10, 19, 20, 79, 91, 99, 126]. As was shown in the Bogalusa Heart Study, excess body weight in childhood has a strong adverse impact on multiple cardiovascular risk factors during adulthood [14, 44, 107, 108].

Autopsy studies have identified atherosclerotic lesions in children as young as 3 years old [15, 112]. Atherosclerosis begins early in life with the appearance of fatty streaks in the aorta during childhood and the coronary arteries in adolescence, so that most young adults have at least a minimal accumulation of these vascular changes. Fatty streaks are potentially reversible, but progression to fibrous plaques, the first step in the development atherosclerosis, may start to develop in young adults 20-30 years old [112]. Known cardiovascular risk factors, such as increased body-mass index (BMI), systolic and diastolic blood pressure, and serum concentrations of total cholesterol (Total-C), triglycerides (TG), low-density lipoprotein cholesterol (LDL-C), and low high-density lipoprotein cholesterol (HDL-C), are strongly associated with the extent of the atherosclerotic lesions [15]. Multiple risk factors cluster in obese people with very high BMI. In children, the normal range for BMI varies with age and sex due to the patterns of growth and development. Approximately 30% of children who have BMI above the 99th percentile have three or more risk factors for cardiovascular disease, independent of age or sex [44].

Noninvasive cardiovascular measurements, such as arterial intimal thickening (IMT) and arterial stiffness, assessed using ultrasound, are significantly increased in obese children [12, 52]. These measurements provide evidence that early, preventable, and reversible detrimental cardiovascular changes are detectable and can be clinically defined in young patients with obesity.

Studies that have tracked overweight children into adulthood indicate that obesity in youth is a significant predictor of adult obesity. Risk factors such as high LDL-C, high systolic blood pressure and high BMI in youth were significantly correlated with carotid artery IMT (higher in obesity) and arterial elasticity (lower in obesity) measured in adulthood [42, 96]. This relationship is true only for overweight children who became obese adults [42, 96]. These and similar findings emphasize the importance of preventing obesity in childhood, since cardiovascular risk in adulthood is predicted by childhood obesity.

METABOLIC SYNDROME

Metabolic syndrome (MetS) was first described in adults as an cluster of risk factors, comprised of obesity associated with insulin resistance, hypertension, dyslipidemia, impaired glucose tolerance and other metabolic changes that carry increased risk of cardiovascular disease [6]. Since the prevalence of obesity has increased in youth, MetS has also begun to become evident at a younger age. Recent estimates suggest that 25-50% of overweight adolescents could be classified as having MetS [24, 68, 73], depending on which criteria are used.

There have been multiple definitions proposed for MetS in children, but the International Diabetes Federation Consensus group is currently the most commonly used definition and is easy to apply in clinical settings [133]. The diagnosis is made if central obesity and two other criteria, listed in Table 1, are present.

**Table 1. Criteria for diagnosis of Metabolic Syndrome
established by the International Diabetes Federation**

Age range (years)	Obesity (Waist Circumference)	Triglycerides (mg/dl)	HDL (mg/dl)	Blood pressure (mmHg)	Glucose (mg/dl)
6-10	>90th percentile				
10-16	>90th percentile or the adult cut-off if lower	≥150	<40	Systolic BP>130 or diastolic BP > 85	>100, or type 2 diabetes
>16 (adult criteria)	WC≥94 cm for males and ≥80 for females	≥150	<40 in males, <50 in females	Systolic BP>130 or diastolic BP > 85	>100, or type 2 diabetes

Metabolic Syndrome is diagnosed if central obesity, based on waist circumference, is present along with two other criteria. Adopted from [133].

Insulin resistance is the main factor in the pathogenesis of MetS and is the result of multiple factors including the accumulation of free fatty acids in the liver, pancreas, fat cells and skeletal muscle, which interfere with the normal insulin signaling [77]. Insulin resistance increases the risk of cardiovascular disease due to alterations in carbohydrate and lipid metabolism, and elevated inflammatory markers Insulin resistance is accentuated during puberty [48].

Dyslipidemia associated with obesity follows a pattern consisting of elevated TG, decreased HDL-C and high normal to mildly elevated LDL-C. Due to insulin resistance, the hepatic availability of nonesterified free fatty acids for TG production is increased [66]. Additionally, TG are converted into small, dense LDL-C and small, dense HDL-C. This is a particularly atherogenic profile, since small, dense LDL-C particles are cleared less effectively by the LDL receptors, which contributes to higher number of such particles remaining in circulation. These small, dense particles have a greater risk of becoming entrapped in the endothelial matrix of the blood vessels. The small, dense HDL-C are less stable and reverse cholesterol transport becomes impaired [23].

Physical activity is part of the lifestyle intervention recommendations for obese children due to the fact that multiple cardiovascular risk factors can be improved. It was shown that a 12-month program of aerobic exercise, in addition to dietary changes, resulted in reduced carotid IMT and increased flow-mediated arterial dilation in previously overweight adolescents [128]. Similar results were demonstrated in another study following 6-months of structured exercise [78]; in that study the improvement in carotid IMT was also associated with favorable changes in BMI, body fat mass, WC, fasting insulin, TG, LDL/HDL ratio and inflammatory markers (C- reactive protein and fibrinogen) [78].

Data from previous exercise studies in adults showed that exercise training effectively decreased circulating TG and increased HDL-C, with no change in LDL-C and Total-C [33]. A meta-analysis of 12 randomized controlled trials performed with children and adolescents 5–19 years of age showed that aerobic exercise typically results in no improvement in Total-C, HDL-C, and LDL-C in children and adolescents, although the analysis was not focused on children with obesity and/or dyslipidemia [59]. However, it has been shown that short-term aerobic exercise results in reduced TG in overweight and obese children, with trends for increased HDL-C [36, 60].

OBESITY AND TYPE 2 DIABETES

Plasma glucose concentration (both fasting and postprandial) is the best predictor for the risk of transitioning from normal glycemic control, to pre-diabetes to type 2 diabetes T2DM [37]. The diagnosis of diabetes was originally based on fasting and postprandial plasma glucose levels; however in 2010 the American Diabetes Association included glycated hemoglobin (HbA1C) as an additional diagnostic criterion. A diagnosis of diabetes in children and adolescents can be made if one or more of the following are present: fasting plasma glucose $\geq$ 126 mg/dl, 2-hour postprandial plasma glucose $\geq$ 200mg/dl, or HbA1C > 6.5% [4]. Pre-diabetes represents a stage of metabolic impairment that precedes the development of diabetes. It is defined as having either impaired fasting glucose (IFG; range = 100-125 mg/dl), or impaired glucose tolerance (IGT; blood glucose concentration two hours after a standard oral glucose challenge in the range of 140-199 mg/dl), or IFT and IGT. The presence of insulin resistance usually precedes the development of T2DM and is characterized by elevated insulin during fasting and/or following carbohydrate ingestion.

Obesity and sedentary lifestyle are major risk factors for developing pre-diabetes and T2DM in children and adults [8, 9, 16, 21]. Overweight children are more likely than their normal weight peers to have insulin resistance, impaired beta-cell function, dyslipidemia, and hypertension [106, 124, 130, 131]. Abdominal adiposity is a strong predictor of insulin resistance [11, 105], which may be mediated, at least in part, by inflammation [54, 113, 114, 126]. A troubling clinical observation is that the progression from insulin resistance to T2DM tends to be faster in adolescents compared to adults [123]. This suggests that insulin resistance and T2DM may require more aggressive treatment in youth compared to adults. This was the conclusion from a recent multi-center trial for adolescents with T2DM, in which half of the study patients could not successfully manage their glycemia with standard medications (metformin with or without rosiglitazone) or home-based lifestyle intervention and had to be placed on insulin therapy within four years of initial diagnosis [132].

GLYCEMIC CONTROL AND GLYCEMIC VARIABILITY

Poor glycemic control in people with diabetes is a risk factor for the development of micro- and macro-vascular complications [30, 31, 111]. Long-term follow-up studies, such as the Diabetes Control and Complications Trial and the UK Prospective Diabetes Study, have demonstrated that tight glycemic control is important for prevention of long-term development of retinopathy, nephropathy, and vascular disease in people with diabetes [2, 3]. Although keeping the average blood glucose under control is intuitively valuable, recent studies have shown that it is more important to avoid acute fluctuations in blood glucose levels in adults with diabetes [82-84]. For example, Monnier et al, reported a positive linear correlation between the mean amplitude of glycemic excursion (MAGE, a calculation of the magnitude of glucose fluctuation) and free radical production [84].

Increased blood glucose fluctuations have been demonstrated in adults who had normal responses during oral glucose tolerance test (OGTT); therefore, glycemic variability may be an early sign of diminishing glucose control and diabetes risk [50]. In a study of adults it was shown that glucose fluctuations gradually increase from normal glucose tolerance (NGT) to IGT to T2DM [120]. It was also shown that increased intra-day glucose variability coincides with the earliest stage of abnormal glucose tolerance [57, 120]. Even though HbA1c is used as a tool for assessing glycemic control and diabetes management, it has failed to fully capture the within- and between-day variability of blood glucose in people with diabetes [25, 76]. The development of continuous glucose monitoring systems (CGMS) has provided an effective tool to measure these fluctuations in glucose concentration at high frequency resolution for several consecutive days. CGMS measures interstitial glucose and the currently available technology has been shown to be a valid and reliable surrogate for blood glucose concentration during glycemic variations [63, 97]. To date, CGMS has been used to study glucose fluctuations in children with type 1 diabetes but has not been used to characterize MAGE in children with T2DM or children at risk for T2DM due to obesity and/or sedentary lifestyle [63, 64].

EXERCISE AND GLYCEMIC CONTROL

The volume of physical activity and level of physical fitness are positively associated with insulin sensitivity and reduced diabetes risk in obese children and adolescents [102].

Studies have shown that glycemic control and insulin sensitivity in adolescents with low physical activity can be significantly improved following a single exercise session and that these beneficial effects last up to 17 hours post-exercise [88, 104]. In untrained adults the effects of single vigorous exercise session on insulin sensitivity and responsiveness was shown to last between 2 and 5 days [80].

The mechanisms that underlie exercise-induced improvement in glucose regulation include increased insulin sensitivity and insulin-independent glucose uptake in skeletal muscle [51]. Exercise training also induces a local contraction-dependent increase in GLUT 4 protein, which enhances the effect of insulin on glucose uptake [28, 29]. For adults with T2DM both endurance and resistive exercise training can lower HbA1c [116] and moderate intensity walking can reduce the amplitude of glucose excursions, measured by CGMS, within 5-7 days [81].

Even in the absence of weight loss, several benefits accrue from regular exercise. Low aerobic fitness is a strong predictor for the presence of metabolic syndrome and cardiovascular disease independent of body fatness in adults [22, 70]. Furthermore, insulin sensitivity is improved in adults in response to exercise training with little or no change in body mass [18, 69, 105].

Likewise, several studies performed with obese adolescents have demonstrated that insulin sensitivity and vascular function increased and hepatic fat content decreased following 8-12 weeks of moderate intensity aerobic exercise even though total body mass fat mass were unchanged [13, 61, 87, 117, 122].

Thus, while reduction in fat mass is an important goal for overweight children, lifestyle interventions that increase physical activity confer significant health benefits on glycemic control independent of weight loss.

OBESITY AND BONE HEALTH

The majority of bone acquisition occurs between the ages of 12-18 years old [98]. Obesity has traditionally been thought to have a protective effect on bone; however, most studies on this subject have been conducted with adults and several recent findings are not in agreement. In theory, increased body mass could act as a positive stimulus on bone because the stress from mechanical loading activates bone turnover, and the increase in adipose tissue is associated with greater production of bone-active hormones and aromatase activity. Leptin is a satiety-regulating hormone produced by the adipose tissue that has been shown to increase the number of osteoblasts and is associated with bone mineral density (BMD) [115, 129]. Aromatase can be found in the adipose tissue and is a key enzyme in the conversion of androgens to estrogens. This enzyme is significant in the bone-fat relationship because estradiol has been associated with obesity in adults [7] and bone accrual in children [62]. Recent studies reported that that there are positive relationships between fat mass and bone mineral content (BMC), but after adjusting for lean mass, these relationships were diminished or no longer present [56, 121]. There is less evidence for how bone metabolism is affected by obesity in children and the story is much less clear compared to what is known for adults. Increased adiposity can result in increased [71], similar [26, 49] or even decreased [46, 100] BMC in children of normal weight. The clinical challenges of examining the growing skeleton in children may account for some of the inconsistencies in the current literature. Maturation is an important factor that must be considered when comparing bone or nearly any other physiological outcome in overweight and normal weight children. Since overweight children tend to progress through puberty at an earlier age the impact of several circulating hormones on bone accrual is also affected [27, 58].

Simple comparisons based on chronological age would result in the erroneous conclusion that obesity per se promotes bone development. Another potential confounding variable in obese children is that lean mass, in addition to fat mass, is greater in overweight children [55, 74]. Lean mass is a major determinate of BMC in children due to the increased mechanical stress placed on the bone.

Consequently, understanding the complex relationship between adipose and bone tissue requires that differences in both lean and fat tissue be considered among normal weight, overweight and obese children [55, 74].

IMPACT OF WEIGHT CHANGE AND EXERCISE
ON BONE HEALTH

Wolff's law states that the bone in a healthy human or animal will adapt to the stresses that are placed upon it [127]. The finding that bone mineral density typically declines during controlled weight-loss in previously obese people supports the importance of bone loading on bone health. One study reported that the rate of BMC reduction was ~11.5 grams per kilogram of fat mass lost [95]. A study of more than 1,000 middle-aged Norwegian women revealed that weight loss accelerates and weight gain decelerates the expected rate of bone loss in the forearm during normal aging [41]. This finding is attributed to the effects of circulating proteins that regulate bone turnover since the mechanical stress on the forearm due to body mass is less than that subjected on the lower body. Studies in previously overweight pre- and postmenopausal women who have lost weight have shown that weight regain does not fully restore BMC or BMD [40, 118]. Importantly, though, when weight loss is achieved only through focused caloric restriction BMD declines in the hip and spine, but if a similar amount of weight is lost through an increase in exercise then BMD at those same sites is not affected [119]. Fewer studies have examined the effect of weight change on adolescents. Studies on adolescents show that BMC may continue to increase even during weight loss, but the weight change through puberty is a strong predictor of change in BMC [101, 110].

The importance of physical activity for bone turnover and function is well established. Physical activities that result in greater bone-loading forces have been shown to be the most beneficial to BMC and BMD. Girls in late adolescence (~17 years old) that participated in rope-skipping had significantly higher bone area in the exercise-loaded bones compared to age-matched girls either participating in soccer or serving as physically-inactive controls [92]. Additionally, prepubertal children that participated in jumping exercises three days per week over seven months had greater increases in BMC than children who performed a similar volume of low- and non-impact exercise [45]. While these studies show the importance of gravitational loading and that high-impact activities are ideal for improving BMD and BMC, it is important to note that low-impact activities should not be discouraged. Compared to adolescent female runners (15-18 years old) BMD is lower in girls who compete at swimming, cycling, or triathlon [32]. However, low-impact activities like cycling and swimming do not appear to be detrimental to bone mass, and their benefit to fitness and cardiometabolic health may outweigh the concern for developing lower BMD. Furthermore, children are encouraged to engage in a variety of physical activities, both weight-bearing and non-weight-bearing.

CONNECTING BONE HEALTH WITH METABOLIC HEALTH

An emerging area of bone research has drawn attention to the interaction between glucose regulation and bone metabolism. Bone tissue was long thought to be an inert storage site for minerals, much like adipose tissue serves as the primary depot for excess lipids, but recent studies have revealed that bone metabolism is integrated with that of other tissues. An example of how this inter-organ communication occurs is the protein, osteocalcin (OC), a bone-specific protein found in circulation that may play a role in glycemic control [5, 38, 39, 67]. OC is produced by osteoblasts and has been used as a marker of bone turnover because it is released into the circulation [94]. The early, rather serendipitous, observation that mice lacking OC become obese and have increased blood glucose and triglycerides sparked interest in the potential role that OC plays outside of the bone [67]. Subsequent studies showed injecting OC into obese mice that are insulin resistant was able to partially restore insulin sensitivity [38]. Additional work in animals and cell cultures demonstrated that OC stimulates insulin release from the pancreas and insulin sensitivity in skeletal muscle [67]. Mice lacking OC had a 50% decrease in β-cells, insulin secreting cells of the pancreas, a 33% decrease in insulin content within the pancreas and decreased expression of insulin target genes within the skeletal muscle [67]. Additionally, in a feed-forward loop, insulin signaling in osteoblasts promotes OC activity [39]. Thus, during increased periods of bone remodeling, such as during growth or in response to exercise, the release of OC from bone to the circulation may offer a mechanism for bone to communicate it's increased metabolic needs and help coordinate the regulation of nutrients among insulin-sensitive tissues.

There is less mechanistic data in humans but many of the studies to date support the association between OC and glucose control. Importantly, and contrary to expectation, obesity, despite having a potential stimulatory effect on bone and OC production, is associated with reduced OC in circulation. For example, in middle school children, total serum OC was negatively related to BMI, total body fat mass, body fat percentage while being positively related to blood glucose [17]. Likewise, OC was 15% lower in prediabetic children compared to age-, weight- and BMI-matched peers [93]. When obese middle-aged men performed a single session of aerobic exercise serum OC increased by 10%, with a concurrent decrease in blood glucose and rise circulating adiponectin, an adipose-derived protein that appears to participate in the cross-talk between bone and adipocytes [72]. To our knowledge there are not yet studies to show whether OC responds a chronic increase in physical activity in adults or children, but it will be important that such studies explore the relationship between changes in OC, pancreatic function, adipocyte-derived proteins, and glycemic regulation. Nevertheless, the existing data have begun to support an important role for bone tissue in whole body nutrient control and that this role may be impaired by obesity in children, but that exercise may potentially restore the effect of bone on glucose metabolism.

CONCLUSION/RECOMMENDATIONS

Childhood obesity and sedentary lifestyle are important public health issues. Lifestyle habits and health risks established in childhood a likely to carry forward into adulthood and have serious personal and socioeconomic impacts. Since many cardiovascular and metabolic risks can be improved by lifestyle changes in childhood, it is increasingly clear that this is a vital period for such interventions. The current American Academy of Pediatrics guidelines for cardiovascular health in childhood recommend lifestyle changes as the primary treatment for pediatric patients who are overweight or obese and have dyslipidemia, but these recommendations can be considered for all of the conditions associated with MetS, T2DM, and obesity. This includes improvement of diet with nutritional counseling and increased physical activity. These guidelines recommend moderate- to- vigorous physical activity for 60 minutes per day for children and adolescents, with emphasis that more intense exercise is necessary 3 days per week. However, it is not specified what volume of exercise should be recommended when specific targets for lipid or glucose control are desired and the effects of exercise on specific lipid, glucose or bone outcomes, independent of weight loss, are unclear.

The current recommendation for physical activity for adults from the American College of Sports Medicine is to achieve 30-60 minutes of moderate-to-vigorous physical activity (MVPA) on ≥5 days per week to maintain or improve cardiometabolic risk, fitness, and body mass [1]. For children the standard recommendation is at least 60 minutes of MVPA per day. In a position statement from the American Diabetes Association issued in

[26] De Schepper J, Van den Broeck M, and Jonckheer MH. Study of lumbar spine bone mineral density in obese children. *Acta Paediatr* 84: 313-315, 1995.

[27] De Simone M, Farello G, Palumbo M, Gentile T, Ciuffreda M, Olioso P, Cinque M, and De Matteis F. Growth charts, growth velocity and bone development in childhood obesity. *Int J Obes Relat Metab Disord* 19: 851-857, 1995.

[28] Dela F, Handberg A, Mikines KJ, Vinten J, and Galbo H. GLUT 4 and insulin receptor binding and kinase activity in trained human muscle. *J Physiol* 469: 615-624, 1993.

[29] Dela F, Mikines KJ, von Linstow M, Secher NH, and Galbo H. Effect of training on insulin-mediated glucose uptake in human muscle. *Am J Physiol* 263: E1134-1143, 1992.

[30] Dinneen S, Gerich J, and Rizza R. Carbohydrate metabolism in non-insulin-dependent diabetes mellitus. *N Engl J Med* 327: 707-713, 1992.

[31] Dinneen SF. The postprandial state: mechanisms of glucose intolerance. *Diabet Med* 14 Suppl 3: S19-24, 1997.

[32] Duncan CS, Blimkie CJ, Cowell CT, Burke ST, Briody JN, and Howman-Giles R. Bone mineral density in adolescent female athletes: relationship to exercise type and muscle strength. *Medicine and science in sports and exercise* 34: 286-294, 2002.

[33] Durstine JL, Grandjean PW, Cox CA, and Thompson PD. Lipids, lipoproteins, and exercise. *Journal of Cardiopulmonary Rehabilitation* 22: 385-398, 2002.

[34] Eaton DK, Kann L, Kinchen S, Shanklin S, Ross JD, Hawkins J, Harris WA, Lowry R, McManus T, Chyen D, Lim C, Whittle L, Brener ND, and Wechsler H. Youth risk behavior serveillance: United States, 2009. *MMWR CDC Surveill Summ* 59: 1-142, 2010.

[35] Eisenmann JC, Welk GJ, Wickel EE, and Blair SN. Stability of variables associated with the metabolic syndrome from adolescence to adulthood: the Aerobics Center Longitudinal Study. *Am J Human Biol* 16: 690-696, 2004.

[36] Ferguson MA, Gutin B, Le NA, Karp W, Litaker M, Humphries M, Okuyama T, Riggs S, and Owens S. Effects of exercise training and its cessation on components of the insulin resistance syndrome in obese children. *International Journal of Obesity and Related Metabolic Disorders: Journal of the International Association for the Study of Obesity* 23: 889-895, 1999.

2012 the recommended amount of exercise for children with T2DM was at least 150 minutes per week [4]. That value, however, represents the minimum needed to have a favorable impact on glycemic control. Since there is considerable inter-individual variability in how specific health outcomes respond to changes in physical activity, and because physical activity impacts nearly all body systems in a favorable manner, we recommend that both children and adults achieve at least 150, and more preferably, 300 minutes per week of MVPA.

ACKNOWLEDGMENTS

The authors are supported by grants from the Endocrine Fellows Foundation, the Department of Pediatrics at the University of Oklahoma Health Sciences Center, the Stanton L. Young Foundation, the Graduate College and the College of Arts and Sciences at the University of Oklahoma, and the National Institutes of Health (Grant number P20 MD000528 from the National Institute on Minority Health and Health Disparities). The views and opinions expressed in this paper are those of the authors.

DISCLOSURE

The authors have no conflicts to declare.

REFERENCES

[1] American College of Sports Medicine. The recommended quantity and quality of exercise for developing and maintaining cardiorespiratory and muscular fitness, and flexibility in healthy adults. *Med Sci Sports Exerc* 30: 975-991, 1998.

[2] UK Prospective Diabetes Study (UKPDS) Group. Effect of intensive blood-glucose control with metformin on complications in overweight patients with type 2 diabetes (UKPDS 34). *Lancet* 352: 854-865, 1998.

[3] The DCCT Research Group. The relationship of glycemic exposure (HbA1c) to the risk of development and progression of retinopathy in the diabetes control and complications trial. *Diabetes* 44: 968-983, 1995.

[4]   American Diabetes Association. Standards of medical care in diabetes--2012. *Diabetes Care* 35 Suppl 1: S11-63, 2012.

[5]   Abseyi N, Siklar Z, Berberoglu M, Hacihamdioglu B, Erdeve SS, and Ocal G. Relationships Between Osteocalcin, GlucoseMetabolism, and Adiponectin in Obese Children:Is there Crosstalk Between Bone Tissue and Glucose Metabolism? *J Clin Res Pediatr Endocrinol* 4: 182-188, 2012.

[6]   Alberti KG, Zimmet P, and Shaw J. Metabolic syndrome--a new world-wide definition. A Consensus Statement from the International Diabetes Federation. *Diabet Med* 23: 469-480, 2006.

[7]   Austin H, Austin JM, Partridge EE, Hatch KD, and Shingleton HM. Endometrial Cancer, Obesity, and Body Fat Distribution. *Cancer Research* 51: 568-572, 1991.

[8]   Bacha F, Gungor N, Lee S, and Arslanian SA. In vivo insulin sensitivity and secretion in obese youth: what are the differences between normal glucose tolerance, impaired glucose tolerance, and type 2 diabetes? *Diabetes Care* 32: 100-105, 2009.

[9]   Bacha F, Lee S, Gungor N, and Arslanian SA. From pre-diabetes to type 2 diabetes in obese youth: pathophysiological characteristics along the spectrum of glucose dysregulation. *Diabetes Care* 33: 2225-2231, 2010.

[10]   Balagopal P, George D, Patton N, Yarandi H, Roberts WL, Bayne E, and Gidding S. Lifestyle-only intervention attenuates the inflammatory state associated with obesity - a randomized controlled study in adolescents. *J Pediatr* 146: 342-348, 2005.

[11]   Basu R, Breda E, Oberg AL, Powell CC, Dalla Man C, Basu A, Vittone JL, Klee GG, Arora P, Jensen MD, Toffolo G, Cobelli C, and Rizza RA. Mechanisms of the age-associated deterioration in glucose tolerance: contribution of alterations in insulin secretion, action, and clearance. *Diabetes* 52: 1738-1748, 2003.

[12]   Beauloye V, Zech F, Tran HT, Clapuyt P, Maes M, and Brichard SM. Determinants of early atherosclerosis in obese children and adolescents. *J Clin Endocrinol Metab* 92: 3025-3032, 2007.

[13]   Bell LM, Watts K, Siafarikas A, Thompson A, Ratnam N, Bulsara M, Finn J, O'Driscoll G, Green DJ, Jones TW, and Davis EA. Exercise alone reduces insulin resistance in obese children independently of changes in body composition. *J Clin Endocrinol Metab* 92: 4230-4235, 2007.

[14]   Berenson GS, Srinivasan SR, Bao W, Newman WP, 3rd, Tracy RE, and Wattigney WA. Association between multiple cardiovascular risk factors and atherosclerosis in children and young adults. The Bogalusa Study. *New England Journal of Medicine* 338: 1650-1656.

[15]   Berenson GS, Srinivasan SR, Bao W, Newman WP, 3rd, Tracy F Wattigney WA. Association between multiple cardiovascular risk and atherosclerosis in children and young adults. The Bogalus Study. *N Engl J Med* 338: 1650-1656, 1998.

[16]   Botero D and Wolfsdorf JI. Diabetes mellitus in childr adolescents. *Arch Med Res* 36: 281-290, 2005.

[17]   Boucher-Berry C, Speiser PW, Carey DE, Shelov SP, Acc Fennoy I, Rapaport R, Espinal Y, and Rosenbaum M. Vita osteocalcin, and risk for adiposity as comorbidities in middle children. *J Bone Miner Res* 27: 283-293, 2012.

[18]   Boule NG, Weisnagel SJ, Lakka TA, Tremblay A, Bergm Rankinen T, Leon AS, Skinner JS, Wilmore JH, Rao DC, and B C. Effects of exercise training on glucose homeostasis: The HEF Family Study. *Diabetes Care* 28: 108-114, 2005.

[19]   Caballero AE, Bousquet-Santos K, Robles-Osorio L, Montag Soodini G, Porramatikul S, Hamdy O, Nobrega ACL, and Ho Overweight Latino children and adolescents have marked en dysfunction and subclinical vascular inflammation in associat excess body fat and insulin resistance. *Diabetes Care* 31: 576-58

[20]   Cali AMG, Zern TL, Taksali SE, de Oliveira AM, Dufour S, C and Caprio S. Intrahepatic fat accumulation and alterations in lip composition in obese adolescents. *Diabetes Care* 30: 3093-3098

[21]   Callahan ST and Mansfield MJ. Type 2 diabetes mellitus in ado *Curr Opin Pediatr* 12: 310-315, 2000.

[22]   Church TS, Finley CE, Earnest CP, Kampert JB, Gibbons LW, SN. Relative associations of fitness and fatness to fibrinoge blood cell count, uric acid and metabolic syndrome. *Int J Ol Metab Disord* 26: 805-813, 2002.

[23]   Cook S and Kavey RE. Dyslipidemia and pediatric obesity. *Pec North Am* 58: 1363-1373, 2011.

[24]   Cowie CC, Rust KF, Ford ES, Eberhardt MS, Byrd-Holt D Williams DE, Gregg EW, Bainbridge KE, Saydah SH, and C Full accounting of diabetes and pre-diabetes in the U.S. Popu 1988-1994 and 2005-2006. *Diabetes Care* 32: 287-294, 2009.

[25]   Dagogo-Jack S. Pitfalls in the use of HbA(1)(c) as a diagnostic ethnic conundrum. *Nat Rev Endocrinol* 6: 589-593, 2010.

[37] Ferrannini E and Camastra S. Relationship between impaired glucose tolerance, non-insulin-dependent diabetes mellitus and obesity. *Eur J Clin Invest* 28 Suppl 2: 3-6; discussion 6-7, 1998.

[38] Ferron M, McKee MD, Levine RL, Ducy P, and Karsenty G. Intermittent injections of osteocalcin improve glucose metabolism and prevent type 2 diabetes in mice. *Bone* 50: 568-575, 2012.

[39] Ferron M, Wei J, Yoshizawa T, Del Fattore A, DePinho RA, Teti A, Ducy P, and Karsenty G. Insulin signaling in osteoblasts integrates bone remodeling and energy metabolism. *Cell* 142: 296-308, 2010.

[40] Fogelholm GM, Sievanen HT, Kukkonen-Harjula TK, and Pasanen ME. Bone mineral density during reduction, maintenance and regain of body weight in premenopausal, obese women. *Osteoporos Int* 12: 199-206, 2001.

[41] Forsmo S, Langhammer A, and Schei B. Past and current weight change and forearm bone loss in middle-aged women: the Nord-Trondelag Health Study, Norway. *Menopause* 16: 1197-1204, 2009.

[42] Freedman DS, Dietz WH, Tang R, Mensah GA, Bond MG, Urbina EM, Srinivasan S, and Berenson GS. The relation of obesity throughout life to carotid intima-media thickness in adulthood: the Bogalusa Heart Study. *Int J Obes Relat Metab Disord* 28: 159-166, 2004.

[43] Freedman DS, Dietz WH, Tang R, Mensah GA, Bond MG, Urbina EM, Srinivasan S, and Berenson GS. The relation of obesity throughout life to carotid intima-media thickness in adulthood: the Bogalusa Heart Study. *Int J Obes Relat Metab Disord* 28: 156-166, 2004.

[44] Freedman DS, Mei Z, Srinivasan SR, Berenson GS, and Dietz WH. Cardiovascular risk factors and excess adiposity among overweight children and adolescents: the Bogalusa Heart Study. *Journal of Pediatrics* 150: 12-17.e12.

[45] Fuchs RK, Bauer JJ, and Snow CM. Jumping improves hip and lumbar spine bone mass in prepubescent children: a randomized controlled trial. *J Bone Miner Res* 16: 148-156, 2001.

[46] Goulding A, Taylor RW, Jones IE, McAuley KA, Manning PJ, and Williams SM. Overweight and obese children have low bone mass and area for their weight. *Int J Obes Relat Metab Disord* 24: 627-632, 2000.

[47] Halcox JPJ, Donald AE, Ellins E, Witte DR, Shipley MJ, Brunner EJ, Marmot MG, and Deanfield JE. Endothelial function predicts progression of carotid intima-media thickness. *Circulation* 119: 1005-1012, 2009.

[48] Hannon TS, Janosky J, and Arslanian SA. Longitudinal study of physiologic insulin resistance and metabolic changes of puberty. *Pediatr Res* 60: 759-763, 2006.

[49] Hasanoglu A, Bideci A, Cinaz P, Tumer L, and Unal S. Bone mineral density in childhood obesity. *J Pediatr Endocrinol Metab* 13: 307-311, 2000.

[50] He LP, Wang C, Zhong L, Yang YZ, Long Y, Zhang XX, Shu SQ, Yu HL, Yu TT, Wang WP, Wang Y, and Ran XW. [Glycemic excursions in people with normal glucose tolerance in Chengdu]. *Sichuan Da Xue Xue Bao Yi Xue Ban* 40: 704-707, 2009.

[51] Holloszy JO. Exercise-induced increase in muscle insulin sensitivity. *J Appl Physiol* 99: 338-343, 2005.

[52] Iannuzzi A, Licenziati MR, Acampora C, Salvatore V, Auriemma L, Romano ML, Panico S, Rubba P, and Trevisan M. Increased carotid intima-media thickness and stiffness in obese children. *Diabetes Care* 27: 2506-2508, 2004.

[53] Ikonomidis I, Stamatelopoulos K, Lekakis J, Vamvakou GD, and Kremastinos DT. Inflammatory and non-invasive vascular markers: the multimarker approach for risk stratification in coronary artery disease. *Atherosclerosis* 199: 3-11, 2008.

[54] Iozzo P. Where does insulin resistance start? The adipose tissue. *Diabetes Care* 32: S168-S173, 2009.

[55] Ivuskans A, Latt E, Maestu J, Saar M, Purge P, Maasalu K, Jurimae T, and Jurimae J. Bone mineral density in 11-13-year-old boys: relative importance of the weight status and body composition factors. *Rheumatol Int*, 2012.

[56] Janicka A, Wren TA, Sanchez MM, Dorey F, Kim PS, Mittelman SD, and Gilsanz V. Fat mass is not beneficial to bone in adolescents and young adults. *J Clin Endocrinol Metab* 92: 143-147, 2007.

[57] Kang Y, Lu JM, Sun JF, Li CL, Wang XL, Zhang XQ, Lu ZH, Dou JT, and Mu YM. [Characteristics of glycemic excursion in different subtypes of impaired glucose intolerance]. *Zhonghua Yi Xue Za Zhi* 89: 669-672, 2009.

[58] Kaplowitz PB, Slora EJ, Wasserman RC, Pedlow SE, and Herman-Giddens ME. Earlier onset of puberty in girls: relation to increased body mass index and race. *Pediatrics* 108: 347-353, 2001.

[59] Kelley GA and Kelley KS. Aerobic exercise and lipids and lipoproteins in children and adolescents: a meta-analysis of randomized controlled trials. *Atherosclerosis* 191: 447-453, 2007.

[60] Kelly AS, Wetzsteon RJ, Kaiser DR, Steinberger J, Bank AJ, and Dengel DR. Inflammation, insulin, and endothelial function in overweight children and adolescents: the role of exercise. *Journal of Pediatrics* 145: 731-736, 2004.

[61] Kelly AS, Wetzsteon RJ, Kaiser DR, Steinberger J, Bank AJ, and Dengel DR. Inflammation, insulin, and endothelial function in overweight children and adolescents: the role of exercise. *J Pediatr* 145: 731-736, 2004.

[62] Klein KO, Larmore KA, de Lancey E, Brown JM, Considine RV, and Hassink SG. Effect of Obesity on Estradiol Level, and Its Relationship to Leptin, Bone Maturation, and Bone Mineral Density in Children. *Journal of Clinical Endocrinology and Metabolism* 83: 3469-3475, 1998.

[63] Klonoff DC. Continuous glucose monitoring: roadmap for 21st century diabetes therapy. *Diabetes Care* 28: 1231-1239, 2005.

[64] Klonoff DC, Buckingham B, Christiansen JS, Montori VM, Tamborlane WV, Vigersky RA, and Wolpert H. Continuous glucose monitoring: an Endocrine Society Clinical Practice Guideline. *J Clin Endocrinol Metab* 96: 2968-2979, 2011.

[65] Koskinen J, Kähönen M, Viikari JS, Taittonen L, Laitinen T, Rönnemaa T, Lehtimäki T, Hutri-Kähönen N, Pietikäinen M, Jokinen E, Helenius H, Mattsson N, Raitakari OT, and Juonala M. Conventional cardiovascular risk factors and metabolic syndrome in predicting carotid intima-media thickness progression in young adults. The Cardiovascular Risk in Young Finns Study. *Circulation* 120: 229-236, 2009.

[66] Laakso M, Sarlund H, and Mykkanen L. Insulin resistance is associated with lipid and lipoprotein abnormalities in subjects with varying degrees of glucose tolerance. *Arteriosclerosis* 10: 223-231, 1990.

[67] Lee NK, Sowa H, Hinoi E, Ferron M, Ahn JD, Confavreux C, Dacquin R, Mee PJ, McKee MD, Jung DY, Zhang Z, Kim JK, Mauvais-Jarvis F, Ducy P, and Karsenty G. Endocrine regulation of energy metabolism by the skeleton. *Cell* 130: 456-469, 2007.

[68] Lee S, Bacha F, Gungor N, and Arslanian S. Comparison of different definitions of pediatric metabolic syndrome: relation to abdominal adiposity, insulin resistance, adiponectin, and inflammatory biomarkers. *J Pediatr* 152: 177-184.e173, 2008.

[69] Lee S, Kuk JL, Davidson LE, Hudson R, Kilpatrick K, Graham TE, and Ross R. Exercise without weight loss is an effective strategy for obesity

reduction in obese individuals with and without type 2 diabetes. *J Appl Physiol* 99: 1220-1225, 2005.

[70] Lee S, Kuk JL, Katzmarzyk PT, Blair SN, Church TS, and Ross R. Cardiorespiratory fitness attenuates metabolic risk independent of abdominal subcutaneous and visceral fat in men. *Diabetes Care* 28: 895-901, 2005.

[71] Leonard MB, Shults J, Wilson BA, Tershakovec AM, and Zemel BS. Obesity during childhood and adolescence augments bone mass and bone dimensions. *The American Journal of Clinical Nutrition* 80: 514-523, 2004.

[72] Levinger I, Zebaze R, Jerums G, Hare DL, Selig S, and Seeman E. The effect of acute exercise on undercarboxylated osteocalcin in obese men. *Osteoporos Int* 22: 1621-1626, 2011.

[73] Li C, Ford ES, Zhao G, and Mokdad AH. Prevalence of pre-diabetes and Its association with clustering of cardiometabolic risk factors and hyperinsulinemia among U.S. adolescents. *Diabetes Care* 32: 342-347, 2009.

[74] Manzoni P, Brambilla P, Pietrobelli A, Beccaria L, Bianchessi A, Mora S, and Chiumello G. Influence of body composition on bone mineral content in children and adolescents. *The American Journal of Clinical Nutrition* 64: 603-607, 1996.

[75] Matthews CE, Chen KY, Freedson PS, Buchowski MS, Beech BM, Pate RR, and Troiano RP. Amount of time spent in sedentary behaviors in the United States, 2003-2004. *Am J Epidemiol* 167: 875-881, 2008.

[76] McCall AL and Kovatchev BP. The median is not the only message: a clinician's perspective on mathematical analysis of glycemic variability and modeling in diabetes mellitus. *J Diabetes Sci Technol* 3: 3-11, 2009.

[77] McGarry JD. *Banting lecture 2001: dysregulation of fatty acid metabolism in the etiology of type 2 diabetes*: Diabetes. 2002 Jan;51(1):7-18.

[78] Meyer AA, Kundt G, Lenschow U, Schuff-Werner P, and Kienast W. Improvement of early vascular changes and cardiovascular risk factors in obese children after a six-month exercise program. *J Am Coll Cardiol* 48: 1865-1870, 2006.

[79] Meyer AA, Kundt G, Steiner M, Schuff-Werner P, and Kienast W. Impaired flow-mediated vasodilation, carotid artery intima-media thickening, and elevated endothelial plasma markers in obese children: the impact of cardiovascular risk factors. *Pediatrics* 117, 2006.

[80] Mikines KJ, Sonne B, Farrell PA, Tronier B, and Galbo H. Effect of physical exercise on sensitivity and responsiveness to insulin in humans. *Am J Physiol* 254: E248-259, 1988.

[81] Mikus CR, Oberlin DJ, Libla J, Boyle LJ, and Thyfault JP. Glycaemic control is improved by 7 days of aerobic exercise training in patients with type 2 diabetes. *Diabetologia* 55: 1417-1423, 2012.

[82] Monnier L and Colette C. Glycemic variability: should we and can we prevent it? *Diabetes Care* 31 Suppl 2: S150-154, 2008.

[83] Monnier L, Colette C, and Owens DR. Glycemic variability: the third component of the dysglycemia in diabetes. Is it important? How to measure it? *J Diabetes Sci Technol* 2: 1094-1100, 2008.

[84] Monnier L, Mas E, Ginet C, Michel F, Villon L, Cristol JP, and Colette C. Activation of oxidative stress by acute glucose fluctuations compared with sustained chronic hyperglycemia in patients with type 2 diabetes. *JAMA* 295: 1681-1687, 2006.

[85] Must A, Jacques PF, Dallal GE, Bajema CJ, and Dietz WH. Long-term morbidity and mortality of overweight adolescents. A follow-up of the Harvard Growth Study of 1922 to 1935. *N Engl J Med* 327: 1350-1355, 1992.

[86] Nader PR, Bradley RH, Houts RM, McRitchie SL, and O'Brien M. Moderate-to-vigorous physical activity from ages 9 to 15 years. *JAMA* 300: 295-305, 2008.

[87] Nassis GP, Papantakou K, Skenderi K, Triandafillopoulou M, Kavouras SA, Yannakoulia M, Chrousos GP, and Sidossis LS. Aerobic exercise training improves insulin sensitivity without changes in body weight, body fat, adiponectin, and inflammatory markers in overweight and obese girls *Metabolism* 54: 1472-1479, 2005.

[88] Nassis GP, Papantakou K, Skenderi K, Triandafillopoulou M, Kavouras SA, Yannakoulia M, Chrousos GP, and Sidossis LS. Aerobic exercise training improves insulin sensitivity without changes in body weight, body fat, adiponectin, and inflammatory markers in overweight and obese girls. *Metabolism* 54: 1472-1479, 2005.

[89] National Center for Health Statistics. Health US. With Special Features on Death and Dying, 2010.

[90] Ogden CL, Carroll MD, Kit BK, and Flegal KM. Prevalence of obesity and trends in body mass index among US children and adolescents, 1999-2010. *Jama* 307: 483-490, 2012.

[91] Peña AS, Wiltshire E, MacKenzie K, Gent R, Piotto L, Hirte C, and Couper J. Vascular endothelial and smooth muscle function relates to

body mass index and glucose in obese and nonobese children. *J Clin Endocrinol Metab* 91: 4467-4471, 2006.

[92] Pettersson U, Nordstrom P, Alfredson H, Henriksson-Larsen K, and Lorentzon R. Effect of high impact activity on bone mass and size in adolescent females: A comparative study between two different types of sports. *Calcif Tissue Int* 67: 207-214, 2000.

[93] Pollock NK, Bernard PJ, Gower BA, Gundberg CM, Wenger K, Misra S, Bassali RW, and Davis CL. Lower uncarboxylated osteocalcin concentrations in children with prediabetes is associated with beta-cell function. *J Clin Endocrinol Metab* 96: E1092-1099, 2011.

[94] Price PA, Parthemore JG, and Deftos LJ. New biochemical marker for bone metabolism. Measurement by radioimmunoassay of bone GLA protein in the plasma of normal subjects and patients with bone disease. *J Clin Invest* 66: 878-883, 1980.

[95] Pritchard JE, Nowson CA, and Wark JD. Bone loss accompanying diet-induced or exercise-induced weight loss: a randomised controlled study. *Int J Obes Relat Metab Disord* 20: 513-520, 1996.

[96] Raitakari OT, Juonala M, and Viikari JS. Obesity in childhood and vascular changes in adulthood: insights into the Cardiovascular Risk in Young Finns Study. *Int J Obes* 29: S101-104, 2005.

[97] Rebrin K, Steil GM, van Antwerp WP, and Mastrototaro JJ. Subcutaneous glucose predicts plasma glucose independent of insulin: implications for continuous monitoring. *Am J Physiol* 277: E561-571, 1999.

[98] Recker RR and Heaney RP. Peak bone mineral density in young women. *Jama* 270: 2926-2927, 1993.

[99] Reinehr T, Kiess W, de Sousa G, Stoffel-Wagner B, and Wunsch R. Intima media thickness in childhood obesity: Relations to inflammatory marker, glucose metabolism, and blood pressure. *Metabolism* 55: 113-118, 2006.

[100] Rocher E, Chappard C, Jaffre C, Benhamou CL, and Courteix D. Bone mineral density in prepubertal obese and control children: relation to body weight, lean mass, and fat mass. *J Bone Miner Metab* 26: 73-78, 2008.

[101] Rourke KM, Brehm BJ, Cassell C, and Sethuraman G. Effect of weight change on bone mass in female adolescents. *J Am Diet Assoc* 103: 369-372, 2003.

[102] Schmitz KH, Jacobs DR, Jr., Hong CP, Steinberger J, Moran A, and Sinaiko AR. Association of physical activity with insulin sensitivity in children. *Int J Obes Relat Metab Disord* 26: 1310-1316, 2002.

[103] Short KR, Blackett PR, Gardner AW, and Copeland KC. Vascular health in children and adolescents: effects of obesity and diabetes. *Vasc Hlth Risk Mgmt* 5: 973-990, 2009.

[104] Short KR, Pratt LV, Teague AM, Man CD, and Cobelli C. Postprandial improvement in insulin sensitivity after a single exercise session in adolescents with low aerobic fitness and physical activity. *Pediatr Diabetes*, 2012.

[105] Short KR, Vittone JL, Bigelow ML, Proctor DN, Rizza RR, Coenen-Schimke JM, and Nair KS. Impact of aerobic training on age-related changes in insulin action and muscle oxidative capacity. *Diabetes* 52: 1888-1896, 2003.

[106] Sinha R, Fisch G, Teague B, Tamborlane WV, Banyas B, Allen K, Savoye M, Rieger V, Taksali S, Barbetta G, Sherwin RS, and Caprio S. Prevalence of impaired glucose tolerance among children and adolescents with marked obesity. *N Engl J Med* 346: 802-810, 2002.

[107] Smoak CG, Burke GL, Webber LS, Harsha DW, Srinivasan SR, and Berenson GS. Relation of obesity to clustering of cardiovascular disease risk factors in children and young adults. The Bogalusa Heart Study. *American journal of epidemiology* 125: 364-372, 1987.

[108] Srinivasan SR, Bao W, Wattigney WA, and Berenson GS. Adolescent overweight is associated with adult overweight and related multiple cardiovascular risk factors: the Bogalusa Heart Study. *Metabolism: Clinical and Experimental* 45: 235-240.

[109] Srinivasan SR, Meyers L, and Berenson GS. Predictability of childhood adiposity and insulin for developing insulin resistance syndrome (syndrome X) in young adulthood: the Bogalusa Heart Study. *Diabetes* 51: 204-209, 2002.

[110] Stettler N, Berkowtiz RI, Cronquist JL, Shults J, Wadden TA, Zemel BS, and Leonard MB. Observational study of bone accretion during successful weight loss in obese adolescents. *Obesity (Silver Spring)* 16: 96-101, 2008.

[111] Stratton IM, Adler AI, Neil HA, Matthews DR, Manley SE, Cull CA, Hadden D, Turner RC, and Holman RR. Association of glycaemia with macrovascular and microvascular complications of type 2 diabetes (UKPDS 35): prospective observational study. *BMJ* 321: 405-412, 2000.

[112] Strong JP, Malcom GT, Newman WP, 3rd, and Oalmann MC. Early lesions of atherosclerosis in childhood and youth: natural history and risk factors. *J Am Coll Nutr* 11: 51S-54S, 1992.

[113] Syrenicz A, Garanty-Bogacka B, Syrenicz M, Gebala A, and Walczak M. Low-grade systemic inflammation and the risk of type 2 diabetes in obese children and adolescents. *Neuro Endocrinol Lett* 27: 435-438, 2006.

[114] Temelkova-Kurktshiev T, Siegert G, Bergmann S, Henkel E, Koehler C, Jaross W, and Hanefeld M. Subclinical inflammation is strongly related to insulin resistance but not to impaired insulin secretion in a high risk population for diabetes. *Metabolism* 51: 743-749, 2002.

[115] Thomas T, Gori F, Khosla S, Jensen MD, Burguera B, and Riggs BL. Leptin acts on human marrow stromal cells to enhance differentiation to osteoblasts and to inhibit differentiation to adipocytes. *Endocrinology* 140: 1630-1638, 1999.

[116] Umpierre D, Ribeiro PAB, Kramer CK, Leitao CB, Zucatti ATN, Azevedo MJ, Gross JL, Ribeiro JP, and Schaan BD. Physical activity advice only or structured exercise training and association with HbA1c levels in type 2 diabetes: a systematic review and meta-analysis. *JAMA* 305: 1790-1799, 2011.

[117] van der Heijden G-J, Toffolo G, Manesso E, Sauer PJJ, and Sunehag AL. Aerobic exercise increases peripheral and hepatic insulin sensitivity in sedentary adolescents. *J Clin Endocrinol Metab* 94: 4292-4299, 2009.

[118] Villalon KL, Gozansky WS, Van Pelt RE, Wolfe P, Jankowski CM, Schwartz RS, and Kohrt WM. A losing battle: weight regain does not restore weight loss-induced bone loss in postmenopausal women. *Obesity (Silver Spring)* 19: 2345-2350, 2011.

[119] Villareal DT, Fontana L, Weiss EP, Racette SB, Steger-May K, Schechtman KB, Klein S, and Holloszy JO. Bone mineral density response to caloric restriction-induced weight loss or exercise-induced weight loss: a randomized controlled trial. *Arch Intern Med* 166: 2502-2510, 2006.

[120] Wang C, Lv L, Yang Y, Chen D, Liu G, Chen L, Song Y, He L, Li X, Tian H, Jia W, and Ran X. Glucose fluctuations in subjects with normal glucose tolerance, impaired glucose regulation and newly diagnosed type 2 diabetes mellitus. *Clin Endocrinol (Oxf)* 76: 810-815, 2012.

[121] Wang MC, Bachrach LK, Van Loan M, Hudes M, Flegal KM, and Crawford PB. The relative contributions of lean tissue mass and fat mass to bone density in young women. *Bone* 37: 474-481, 2005.

[122] Watts K, Beye P, Siafarikas A, Davis EA, Jones TW, O'Driscoll G, and Green DJ. Exercise training normalizes vascular dysfunction and improves central adiposity in obese adolescents. *J Am Coll Cardiol* 43: 1823-1827, 2004.

[123] Weiss R and Caprio S. The metabolic consequences of childhood obesity. *Best Pract Res Clin Endocrinol Metab* 19: 405-419, 2005.

[124] Williams DE, Caldwell BL, Cheng YJ, Cowie CC, Gregg EW, Geiss LS, Engelgau MM, Narayan KM, and Imperatore G. Prevalence of impaired fasting glucose and its relationship with cardiovascular disease risk factors in US adolescents, 1999-2000. *Pediatrics* 116: 1122-1126, 2005.

[125] Wilson PW, D'Agostino RB, Sullivan L, Parise H, and Kannel WB. Overweight and obesity as determinants of cardiovascular risk: the Framingham experience. *Arch Intern Med* 162: 1867-1872, 2002.

[126] Winer JC, Zern TL, Taksali SE, Dziura J, Cali AM, Wollschlager M, Seyal AA, Weiss R, Burgert TS, and Caprio S. Adiponectin in childhood and adolescent obesity and its association with inflammatory markers and components of the metabolic syndrome. *J Clin Endocrinol Metab* 91: 4415-4423, 2006.

[127] Wolff J, Maquet PGJ, and Furlong R. *The law of bone remodelling.* Berlin ; London: Springer-Verlag, 1986.

[128] Woo KS, Chook P, Yu CW, Sung RY, Qiao M, Leung SS, Lam CW, Metreweli C, and Celermajer DS. Effects of diet and exercise on obesity-related vascular dysfunction in children. *Circulation* 109: 1981-1986, 2004.

[129] Yamauchi M, Sugimoto T, Yamaguchi T, Nakaoka D, Kanzawa M, Yano S, Ozuru R, Sugishita T, and Chihara K. Plasma leptin concentrations are associated with bone mineral density and the presence of vertebral fractures in postmenopausal women. *Clin Endocrinol (Oxf)* 55: 341-347, 2001.

[130] Yeckel CW, Taksali S, Dziura J, Weiss R, Burgert TS, Sherwin RS, Tamborlane WV, and Caprio S. The normal glucose tolerance continuum in obese youth: evidence for impairment in beta-cell function independent of insulin resistance. *J Clin Endocrinol Metab* 90: 747-754, 2005.

[131] Yeckel CW, Weiss R, Dziura J, Taksali S, Dufour S, Burgert TS, Tamborlane WV, and Caprio S. Validation of insulin sensitivity indices from oral glucose tolerance test parameters in obese children and adolescents. *J Clin Endocrinol Metab* 89: 1096-1101, 2004.

[132] Zeitler P, Hirst K, Pyle L, Linder B, Copeland K, Arslanian S, Cuttler L, Nathan DM, Tollefsen S, Wilfley D, and Kaufman F. A clinical trial to maintain glycemic control in youth with type 2 diabetes. *N Engl J Med* 366: 2247-2256, 2012.

[133] Zimmet P, Alberti KG, Kaufman F, Tajima N, Silink M, Arslanian S, Wong G, Bennett P, Shaw J, and Caprio S. The metabolic syndrome in children and adolescents - an IDF consensus report. *Pediatr Diabetes* 8: 299-306, 2007.

In: Childhood Obesity   ISBN: 978-1-62618-874-7
Editor: Callum G. Jackson   © 2013 Nova Science Publishers, Inc.

Chapter 3

CONTRIBUTORY INFLUENCES PROMOTING CHILDHOOD ADIPOSITY IN A MEDITERRANEAN ISLAND POPULATION

S. Savona-Ventura[1,*], C. Scerri[2,†] and C. Savona-Ventura[3,‡]

[1]Department of Education, University of Malta, Malta
[2]Department of Health, Malta
[3]University of Malta Medical School, Malta

ABSTRACT

The Maltese population is a small island population in the Central Mediterranean. The nutritional concerns relating to Maltese children in the mid-twentieth century were primarily those relating to undernutrition and insufficient body weight when compared to their British counterparts. There has been in the last decades a shift in the childhood weight concerns with the observation of an alarming rise in childhood adiposity reaching to 28.8% and 32.7% in 5-year old body and girls respectively; and 48.9% and 45.1% respectively at 9 years of age. The underlying cause for this rise has been shown to be partly related to perinatal and

* E-mail: steffi.savona@gmail.com.
† E-mail: christopher_scerri@hotmail.com.
‡ E-mail: charles.savona-ventura@um.edu.mt..

early childhood feeding programming that appears to offset any later attempts to control for later childhood adiposity. A further association has been described for childhood adiposity to an increased mean passive activity time with a corresponding negative association to mean active physical activity and sleeping times. Transgenerational associations towards a familiar tendency to adiposity have been observed these possibly being related to the family's socio-economic status or a family history of metabolic syndrome components. It is advised that parents of children at risk – low or high birth weight; bottle fed children; early childhood obesity – should be regularly advised actively regarding health lifestyle and nutrition options. The observed relationship between childhood adiposity to the combination of decreased physical activity and increased energy-dense foods suggests that life-style intervention could have a possible positive influence in decreasing the problems of childhood adiposity.

INTRODUCTION

Adiposity has become a worldwide concern, targeting particularly the developed world. Studies have indicated that "obesity begets obesity", so that children of obese parents are at a greater risk of developing obesity throughout their life [Birth and Fisher, 1998]. This familiar relationship of adiposity suggests that obesity may be explained in part by a genetic or hereditary element [Bouchard, 1991]. The genetic element may in fact interact synergistically with the physical and social environment, influenced by parenting attitudes, to produce the observed hereditary relationship [Johnson and Birch, 1994]. A detailed understanding of the interrelationship between the genetic and environmental factors is essential to enable in the design of effective preventive interventions [Birch and Fisher, 1998].

The prevalence of childhood adiposity is rapidly growing worldwide and has reached alarming rates. Many of those individuals who develop obesity in childhood will remain obese in adulthood. Guo and Chumlea [1999] suggested that the probability of childhood obesity persisting into adulthood increases by 20% at 4 years of age and to 80% by adolescence. Childhood obesity has been shown to have long term effects on mortality and morbidity [Wang and Lobstein, 2006], so that more than 60% of overweight children have at least one additional risk factor for cardiovascular disease such as raised blood pressure, hyperlipidaemia or hyperinsulinaemia [Dietz, 2001]. In addition, most cases of Type 2 diabetes in children and adolescents are attributed to obesity [Fagot-Campagna et al. 2000]. In the light of these findings, prevention of adiposity in children has been argued as a priority for public health researchers to combat the adult obesity epidemic [Muller et al. 2001].

The increased prevalence of adiposity and the associated diabetic condition in the Maltese adult population started receiving the attention of the Maltese public health authorities in the 1950s [Galea, 1958]. There has been since a further increase in adiposity prevalence over the last decades – an increase that has further extended to the child and adolescent population. The 2001-2002 Health Behaviour in School-children Study [HSBC] showed that Maltese children have very high levels of adiposity being even higher than those reported for the United States. The study showed that the prevalence of adiposity in Maltese children was 33.3%; marginally higher than the 31.9% figure reported for American children [Janssen et al. 2005]. Maltese children also had the highest adiposity rates in the European Union [Lobstein et al. 2004]. Since childhood obesity is a precursor of adult obesity with the associated co-morbidities, it is essential that a clear understanding of the biological mechanisms behind this developing epidemic are understood in order that targeted life-style changes may be timely introduced.

STUDY POPULATION CHARACTERISTICS

The Maltese population is a small island community situated in the central Mediterranean that has been identified as having particular geographical and cultural stressors that can influence the risk for developing a spectrum of metabolic disease including diabetes and obesity [Formosa et al. 2012]. With a land mass of only 316 km^2 and a total population in 2011 of 416,110 persons, the community has one of the highest population densities worldwide [1317 per km^2] [N.S.O., 2012].

The overall health of the Maltese population is presently consistent with that of a developed country with a life expectancy in 2010 of 83.1 years in females and 78.9 years in males. The crude birth rate stands at 10.3 per 1000 population, the crude death rate at 7.9 per 1000 population. Dietary changes associated with a higher standard of living have contributed to making the metabolic syndrome the primary health problem of the population. Adiposity with a BMI $\geq$25 kg/m^2[aged 25 to 64 years – men 76.8%, women 54.9%]; hyperglycaemia of $\geq$7.0 mmol/l [aged $\geq$18 years – men 9.0%, women 10.7%]; hypercholesterolemia [aged 25-64 years – men 68.8%, women 56.1%] and hypertension [aged 25-64 years – men 33.1%, women 31.4%] are all common conditions. Long term complications from these conditions [e.g. coronary heart disease and stroke] cause 38.3% of all deaths [N.S.O., 2011; D.H.I.R., 2012]. The obesity co-morbidities are expected to increase progressively in line with the observed increase in childhood obesity.

The 1981 WHO National Diabetes Study had shown that the Maltese has significant risk criteria for developing type 2 diabetes mellitus and its co-morbidities [Katona et al. 1983]. A familiar tendency to the disease was noted suggesting a possible genetic contributor; though in the female population statistical significance for the familiar inter-relationship was noted with the individual's mother and siblings, but not the father suggesting an intrauterine environment modulation of risk [Savona-Ventura et al. 2003]. A number of molecular SNPlotypes representing inflammatory response, metabolic syndrome and MODY genes have been identified in the Maltese population as potential contributors towards an increased risk to developing Type 2 diabetes mellitus. However, this SNPlotype profile showed no statistically significant differences when compared to a comparative Libyan population, suggesting a similar genetic profile in relation to these disorders in these two populations [Al-Asthar, 2009]. This is not surprising since, in spite of being a small island population, its situation has ensured a varied genetic intermix involving circum-Mediterranean and European populations [Formosa et al. 2012].

CHILDHOOD ADIPOSITY IN MALTA

The problem of childhood obesity in Malta seems to have come to the fore only in the latter part of the twentieth century. In the mid-20th century, child nutrition was already a topical concern of the public health authorities in Malta. The issue then, however, was not one of over-nutrition, but rather of under-nutrition. During 1949, a survey of 15468 children aged 5-14 years revealed that 7.2% of the children were in a bad or poor state of nutrition, while a further 14.3% were reported as being in a fair or slightly sub-normal state. At 5 years of age the mean body weight of Maltese children was just below the 50th percentile when compared to the British percentile weight standards for boys and girls. By 9 years of age, the mean body weight was around the 25th percentile; while at 14 years of age, the mean body weight for both genders was around the 10th percentile. The comparative fall in mean body weight of Maltese children with age compared to their British counterparts suggests that while childhood nutrition in Maltese children in 1949 may have been nearly comparable to 1965 British standards until the age of five years; nutritional standards appeared to deteriorate in the subsequent childhood years thus affecting growth and physical development (Figure 1). The prime concern for the public health authorities then was the promotion of better nutrition practices [Savona-Ventura and Scerri, in press]. Serious efforts were made by the Maltese health authorities to address infant and child health in the subsequent years with impressive results, turning the tide and eventually shifting within three decades the nutritional concerns in children from under-nutrition to over-nutrition. By 1956, only 9.4% of children were reported to be in a fair or bad state of nutrition, even though the mean weights at age 14-15 years were still below the U.K. 20th centile [Galea, 1958].

In 1981, the WHO National Diabetes Program led an epidemiological study to assess the prevalence of diabetes and co-morbidities in the Maltese population aged >15 years. The survey established that the mean Body Mass Index was in the higher range of normal at 22.8 kg/m^2 in males and 23.0 in females aged 15-24 years, but in the just overweight range in individuals aged 25-34 years [male 25.6; females 25.3] [Katona et al. 1983].

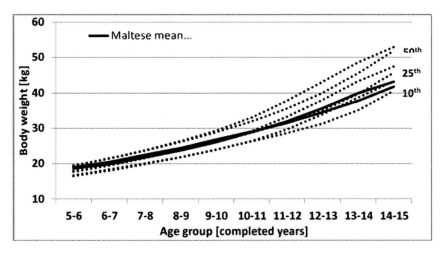

Figure 1. Body weight distribution by age and gender of Maltese Children in 1949 compared to 1960 British children centile weight charts.

Maltese young adults presenting with a pregnancy during the period 1998-2006, exhibited an increasing pre-pregnancy BMI with increasing age from 23.2 + 4.3 kg/m2 [n = 250] in those aged 14-16 years, to 24.2 + 4.7 [n = 1150] in those aged 17-19 years, and 25.3 + 5.2 [n = 4648] in those women aged 20-24 years (Figure 2). The mean pre-pregnancy BMI progressively increased with increasing maternal age [unpublished data–National Obstetric

Information System data base held by the Department of Health Information and Research, Malta].

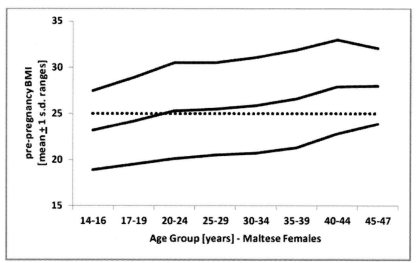

Figure 2. Mean + standard deviation Body Mass Index distribution by age in Maltese female population aged 14-47 years: 1998-2006 [unpublished data, NOIS data base].

The concerns that childhood adiposity had become an important public health issue in the Maltese population were confirmed by subsequent studies. A point prevalence study carried out in 1991 on Maltese children showed that obesity, defined as a value higher that the 97th weight-for-height percentile, was about 12% at 5 years of age [boys 13.0%, girls 11.5%] and 22% at 10 years of age [boys 18.9%, girls 24.3%] [Galea et al. 1992]. A study comparing adiposity rates among European Union countries carried out by the International Obesity Task Force [Lobstein et al. 2004] showed that Maltese children aged 7-11 years topped the adiposity [overweight/obese] rate with figures of 32.7% of boys and 38.5% of girls. The obesity rate was reported to be about 12%. A high adiposity rate [overweight 25.4%, obese 7.9%] was also reported in Maltese adolescents aged 10-16 years [boys 30.9%, girls 20.1%]. These reported rates in Maltese youths were closely followed by those in comparative youths from the United States of America [Janssen et al. 2005]. High childhood obesity rates for Maltese children have been confirmed at all age groups in subsequent studies. A longitudinal follow-up study of a cohort of 3435 children born in 2001 showed that the adiposity rate at six years of age was 40.1% in boys and 31.5% in girls. The same cohort reassessed three years later showed higher adiposity rates at 47.9% and 39.5% respectively.

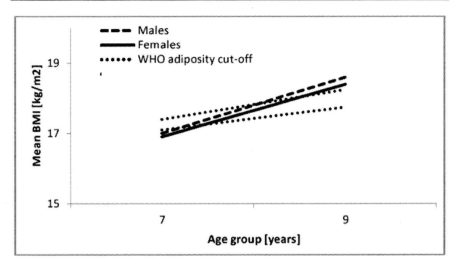

Figure 3. Mean Body Mass Index distribution by age in Maltese population aged 7 and 9 years: child cohort born 2001 [after Farrugia Sant'Angelo and Grech, 2011].

While at seven years of age the mean BMI was just below the adiposity cut-off values for both genders, the mean BMI at 9 years of age had gone over the cut-off BMI values for that age in both genders (Figure 3) [Farrugia Sant'Angelo and Grech, 2011]. There is no doubt that the problem has now shifted from that of under-nutrition in the mid-twentieth century to one of over-nutrition at the beginning of the twenty-first century. Since no significant changes have affected the population gene pool in the last decades, the reasons for this shift must have been dependant on lifestyle and nutritional changes over the last decades.

BIRTH WEIGHT INFLUENCES

Intrauterine nutrition has been shown through metabolic programming or imprinting to influence the risks of developing obesity and other comorbidities of the metabolic syndrome [Barker, 1998; Waterland and Garza, 1999]. The environmental factors of under-nutrition during intrauterine life modulate the individual's epigenetic switches allowing him/her to deal with future starvation. Similarly, intrauterine over-nutrition initiates developmental changes that in adulthood predispose to adiposity and other features of the metabolic syndrome. Nutritional intrauterine starvation during the last trimester of pregnancy and the first months of life caused by the Dutch famine of 1994-45 has been demonstrated to be related to lower obesity prevalence rates. However, exposure during the first half of pregnancy was associated with higher obesity prevalence than in non-exposed controls [Ravelli et al. 1976]. A later follow-up study of the same cohort of individuals now aged 50 years showed that those females exposed to intrauterine starvation had higher BMI levels that non-exposed woman. There were no significant differences between famine-exposed or non-exposed men [Ravelli et al. 1999]. In the Pima Indian population, children born to women suffering from gestational diabetes and hence presumably overfed in utero had higher risks for childhood obesity than those born to women with a normal carbohydrate metabolic profile. This difference persisted after correction for other influencing factors [Pettit et al. 1983]. In the Maltese adult population, a definite correlation has been demonstrated between low and high birth weight and the subsequent risk of developing gestational diabetes mellitus [Savona-Ventura and Chircop, 2003]. A similar correlation has been shown between low and high birth weights and the risk for developing childhood obesity (Figure 4). This latter study showed that, at five years of age, there is a definite statistically increased risk of having childhood adiposity in those children born macrosomic, but while the risk was higher in those born of low birth weight the difference was not statistically significant.

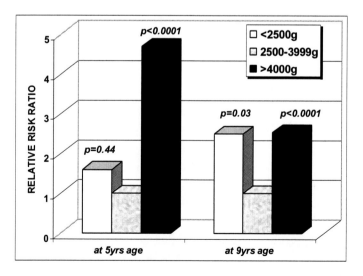

Figure 4. Relative risk for childhood obesity by birth weight at 5 and 9 years of age, [after Scerri and Savona-Ventura, 2010].

A statistically significant increase in adiposity risk was shown in both low and high birth weight children at nine years of age [Scerri and Savona-Ventura, 2010].

Intrauterine starvation sets up a vicious cycle whereby intrauterine nutritionally deprived individuals predispose to the subsequent development of metabolic abnormalities through the Barker cycle and thus in their turn contribute to intrauterine over-nutrition in their subsequent children though the Pedersen cycle (Figure 5) [Savona-Ventura, 2006; Formosa et al. 2012]. This cycle of metabolic modulation has been demonstrated in Maltese women born during the siege condition of the Second World War where women born during the siege period were shown to have infants with statistically higher birth weights than their counterparts born before and after the siege [Savona-Ventura et al. 2007]. There has been a progressive statistically significant change [P<0.0001] in birth weights of Maltese infants over the last decades exhibiting an overall drop since the 1950s with an increase in low birth weight infants [3.3% to 7.8%] and a decrease in macrosomia [18.4% to 4.4%].

It appears that overall the proportion of low and high birth weight infants at risk of foetal origins for adult-onset disease has decreased from 21.7% to 12.2% (Table 1) [Agius et al. 1966; Grech and Savona-Ventura, 1988; Zammit et al., 2010]. The increase in childhood obesity rates over the same period suggests that while intrauterine nutrition may play a role, subsequent lifestyle practices relating to nutrition and physical exercise may be more relevant players.

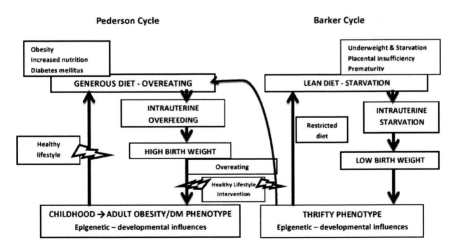

Figure 5. Barker – Pederson Cycles.

Table 1. Birth weight characteristics: Maltese births 1951 and 2009

Year	1951-59	1981	2009
Birth weight [mean + s.d.]	3375 + 621 gm.	3356 + 525 gm.	3252 + 516 gm.
Number of births	4103	4558	4146
% total national births	5.2%	87%	100%
% birth weight <2.5 kg	3.3%	3.6%	7.8%
% birth weight >4.0 kg	18.4%	10.2%	4.4%

DIETARY CONTRIBUTORS

Intrauterine nutrition as reflected by the infant birth weight has been shown to be an important determinant for the risks for eventual childhood adiposity. This appears to be further influenced by postnatal feeding during infanthood.

In a cross-sectional survey of 9,357 German children entering school, the prevalence of obesity in children who had never been breast-fed was 1.6-fold higher than in previously breast-fed children. A clear dose-response effect of the duration of breast-feeding on the prevalence of later obesity emerged from this study. The protective effect of breast-feeding was not attributable to differences in social class or lifestyle. After adjustment for potential confounding factors, the study found that breast-feeding remained a protective factor against the development of overweight and obesity [von Kries et al, 1999].

The interrelationship between type of infant feeding and childhood adiposity in Maltese children aged five years was demonstrated in a recent study. The study, carried out on a cohort of 206 Maltese five-year-old children, confirmed that breast-fed children showed a statistically significant lower prevalence of adiposity when compare to artificially-fed ones. This inter-relationship was also evident at nine years of age but statistical significance was not reached in this later cohort of 230 children (Figure 6). The loss of statistical strength was attributed to the possibility that the introduction of other influencing factors, such as diet and lack of physical exercise, may have modified the metabolic imprinting generated by artificial-feeding [Scerri and Savona-Ventura, 2011].

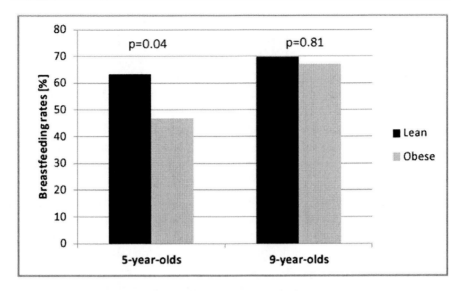

Figure 6. Breastfeeding rates in lean and obese Maltese children [after Scerri and Savona-Ventura, 2011].

Breastfeeding rates in the Maltese Islands have seen a definite shift throughout the last thirty decades with an overall rise in initial breast-feeding rates from 24.5% in 1980 to 56.1% in 2010 [Savona-Ventura and Grech, 1990; D.H.I.R., 1999-2010]. While there appears to have been a general increase in initial breast-feeding rates, this effort is not generally maintained and, in 2000, as much as 55% of initial breastfeeding mothers opted to shift to artificial feeding within the first month of the infant's life [Attard Montalto, 2002]. This high drop-out rate persists to date in spite of the social services support available to working mothers.

The initiation of artificial feeding in a child's life heralds the onset of a pattern of unhealthy nutritional practices that often persist in adulthood. Dietary habits and food preferences, caloric content of the diet, and nutrient composition all appear to modulate the risk of obesity development. People's eating habits have changed significantly in recent decades. Globally the amount of food available has risen over time. On average, a woman needs to consume 2000 calories a day to maintain her weight, and the figure for men is 2500 calories. In 1961, the number of calories available per person per day was 2300. This has risen to 2800 calories by 1988 and is likely to exceed 3000 by around 2015. Also, food prices have fallen over time – the real price of rice, wheat, maize, fat and sugar fell by about 60% between 1960 and 2000. At the beginning of the 20th century, people ate less than 5 kg of sugar per year. In

Europe today, this has risen to 40 - 60 kg. At the same time, people are not eating enough fruit and vegetables [W.H.O., 2006]. Worldwide restaurant food consumption increased considerably in children and adults between 1977 and 1996. The proportion of foods that children consumed from restaurants and fast food outlets increased by nearly 300% during that 19 year period [Johnson-Tayloy and Everhart, 2006]. Portion sizes in restaurants increased from 1970 to 1999 with the result that soft drinks contain an additional 206 kJ, hamburger 407 kJ, and French fries 286 kJ [Young and Nestle, 2002]. In a longitudinal study of 101 girls aged 8-12 years, the frequency of eating quick-service food at base line was associated with changes in BMI z scores at 11-year and 19-year follow-up [Thompson et al. 2004]. A further study has suggested that, over a 1-year period, children who consume fried foods away from home more frequently were heavier and had greater total energy intake, compared with children with low frequency of fried food consumption away from home [Taveras et al. 2005]. Sweetened beverage consumption and its possible association with the increased prevalence of overweight and obesity among children have been assessed in various studies. The Bogalusa Heart study examined energy intake among 10-year-old children from 1973 to 1994 and findings from the study showed that children who did not consume sweetened beverages did not have increased energy intake. However, energy intake did increase among children who consumed small to moderate to large amounts of sweetened beverages [Nicklas et al. 2001]. In a pilot intervention study, Ebbeling et al. [2006] showed that reducing sweetened beverage consumption reduced body weight in adolescents in the upper baseline BMI tertile. Interestingly Janssen et al. [2005] when considering intake of soft drinks in 34 [primarily European] countries did not find any association with overweight status.

Until the early twentieth century, the diet in Malta was the same for the general population, especially for the lower socio-economic classes. The majority of the population consumed large quantities of barley bread and wine together with olives, oil, onions, garlic, cheese and very little fish or meat, since meat was rarely affordable. They also consumed seasonal fruit and vegetables in abundance. In the latter half of the twentieth century, the financial status and social conditions for the Maltese population improved greatly leading to an alteration in the dietary habits concentrating on the high consumption of food high in fats and carbohydrates such as fried eggs, bacon and chips [Cassar, 1988]. Nutritional studies carried out in 1981 confirmed that the Maltese consume large amounts of food with a large proportion of fat [43.5-47.7%], starch [25.4-20.4%], and sugar [14.9-14.8%] [Katona et al,

1983]. Thus the Maltese diet has changed from one that was high in complex carbohydrates and low in fats, especially animal fats, to one that is low in complex carbohydrates and high in refined carbohydrate [sugar and starch] intake and high in total fats, especially animal fats. A recent nutritional survey carried out among young adults aged 18-26 years showed that the mean and standard deviation general diet score reflecting the frequency of resorting to health and unhealthy snacks, drinks, meals, and type of food preparation was 0.46 + 1.02. This is far below the ideal score of five reflecting very health dietary habits behaviour [a minus five score reflects very unhealthy dietary habits behaviour] [Savona-Ventura, 2012]. The tendency towards less-than-ideal dietary habits in young adults aged 18-24 years is further outlined by the 2007 Lifestyle Survey (Table 2) conducted among a cohort of 37,522 individuals. In the same study, 29.8% of the study population visited restaurants at least once a month. In contrast, only 4.5% attended live sport events on an approximate monthly as a leisure activity [N.S.O., 2009].

Unhealthy nutritional habits in young adults are initiated in childhood. A recent nutritional survey carried out among a cohort of five-year old Maltese children whose overall adiposity rate was 30.8% [boys 28.8%, girls 32.7%] showed that parents of adipose children reported different nutritional habits than those reported by parents of lean children.

Table 2. Lifestyle Survey data relevant to obesity – Maltese population aged 18-24 years: 2007

Lifestyle factors	Males N = 20385	Females N = 17137	Total N = 37522
Follow a particular diet	4760 (23.4%)	7677 (44.8%)	12437 (34.1%)
Do not consume fruit	3183 (15.6%)	1643 (9.6%)	4826 (12.6%)
Do not consume vegetables	1881 (9.2%)	861 (5.0%)	2742 (7.1%)
Do not consume fried foods	992 (4.9%)	3812 (22.2%)	4804 (13.6%)
Do not drink any form of alcohol	3316 (16.3%)	6002 (35.0%)	9318 (25.6%)
Do not drink wine	9990 49.0%)	9054 (52.8%)	19044 (50.8%)
Do not drink beer	7743 (38.0%)	16121 (94.1%)	23884 (63.6%)
Do not drink spirit alcohol	9457 (46.4%)	9096 (53.1%)	18553 (49.7%)
Do not walk for at least 30 minutes per week	11351 (55.7%)	7411 (43.2%)	18762 (49.5%)
Do not do any intensive exercise	9293 (45.6%)	9872 (57.6%)	19165 (51.6%)
Do not attend a gym/fitness club at least once weekly	16478 (80.8%)	14524 (84.8%)	31002 (82.8%)

The former appeared to more frequently partake energy-rich foods including more frequent consumption of meat/fish and potato chips. They also more frequently resorted to fruit juices/soft drinks and milk. They were less likely to consume fresh fruit/vegetables, milk products such as cheese/yogurt, and sweets/biscuits. None of the reported differences were however statistically significant. The reported dietary habits in a cohort of nine-year-old children with an overall adiposity rate of 47.0% [boys 48.9%, girls 45.1%] showed different patterns. The adipose children consumed fresh fruit/vegetables, cheese and fish more frequently than their lean counterparts. In contrast they consumed less fruit juices/soft drinks, milk or yogurt, meat, chips and sweets/biscuits. The changes in dietary habits noted in the two cohorts suggest that definite efforts were being made by the parents of adipose children to deliberately restrict sweet intake and the consumption of energy dense foods in order to control the child's weight [Scerri and Savona-Ventura, 2011]. It is likely, however, that the adipose children at nine-years of age have through intrauterine and early childhood nutrition modulation already attained their predisposition towards adulthood adiposity, especially when associated with the general lack of physical exercise. This would suggest that early intervention with lifestyle modifications must in high risk infants be made early in infant and early childhood.

PHYSICAL EXERCISE

The degree of a person's physical activity markedly affects total energy expenditure and thus energy balance. Low physical activity levels are associated with obesity in children and adolescents, and may be both the cause and consequence of increased weight [Klesges et al. 1995]. Although young people are more physically active than adults, the worldwide increase in overweight among youth has raised concerns about the adequacy of habitual activity in children and adolescents. Societal changes such as increased car ownership, unfriendly walking and cycling environments, and increasing choices in electronic entertainment, combined with the concern about increased weight, have created a need to understand physical activity trends in youth. In some studies, the obesity risk of a child has been correlated to time spent viewing television, that is, times with low level of physical activity and low energy expenditure. The relation of overweight and obesity to physical activity, television viewing time, and videogame playing was studied in 7-9-year-old Portuguese children [Carvalhal et al. 2007]. Eating while watching

Table 4. Three generation relationships of BMI and birth weights [after Agius et al. in prep.]

1st generation	BMI <25 kg/m2		BMI >25 kg/m2	
2nd generation Birth weight [kg] Adult BMI [kg/m2]	3.16 + 0.46 22.69 + 4.21		3.40 + 0.52 24.83 + 4.40	
	BMI <25 kg/m2	BMI >25 kg/m2	BMI <25 kg/m2	BMI >25 kg/m2
3rd generation BW [kg]	2.93 + 0.57	3.31 + 0.41	3.07 + 0.42	3.37 + 0.46

The familiar, apparently hereditable, predisposition towards adiposity may however not necessarily be simply a direct relationship to genetic predisposition. The genetic predisposition may interact synergistically with the physical and social environment of the family, influenced by parenting attitudes, to produce the observed apparently inherited patterns of adiposity within families [Costanzo and Woody, 1985 as cited in Johnson and Birch, 1994]. There is no doubt that the dietary habits of children and adolescents are influenced by parents and other household members [Birch and Fisher, 1998]. This influence may be tempered by food-type availability determined by socio-economic and other factors.

Children and adolescents of lower socioeconomic status have been reported to be less likely to eat fruits and vegetables, and to have a higher intake of total and saturated fat [Sobal and Stunkard, 1989]. In addition, physical activity level of children was also found to be related to socioeconomic status and living conditions, peer pressure, and the degree of physical activity of the parents [Klesges RC et al. 1993]. The unhealthy lifestyle predisposed to by the socioeconomic status of the family would contribute towards childhood and subsequent adulthood adiposity. Food insecurity may contribute to the inverse relationship of obesity prevalence with socioeconomic status, but the relationship is a complex one [Alaimo et al. 2001]. Other barriers which low income families may face are lack of safe places for physical activity and lack of consistent access to healthful food choices, particularly fruits and vegetables. Low cognitive stimulation in the home, low socioeconomic status, and maternal obesity all predict development of obesity [Strauss and Knight, 1999].

An inter-relationship between childhood adiposity and socio-economic status was observed in Maltese children. The mean Body Mass Index of 6-

TV appeared to be common practice among Portuguese families. In contrast, computer use required a more centred focus of attention and the use of both hands so that eating snacks, while playing on the computer takes place during small breaks between the different games or change of level of difficulty. To support this, no association was found regarding the time children use the computer with the BMI or obesity. The average mean values for BMI were higher for both boys and girls that did not practice physical education while most boys and girls spent between 4 to 6 hours watching TV. The mean values for BMI rose as the hours that both boys and girls spent watching TV; playing electronic games and computer use. The prevalence of obesity rose as the hours of watching TV increased. The highest prevalence recorded was for boys [32.5%] and girls [32.5%] that watched TV for 4 to 6 hours per day. In the obesity review based on the WHO's 2001-2002 HBSC study, Janssen et al. [2005] found that within most countries physical activity levels were lower and television viewing times were higher in overweight compared to normal weight youth. Similar observations were made by the Third National Health and Nutrition Examination survey [NHANES III] 1988-1994, where the collected data of 4096 US children aged 8 to 16 years was examined. This found that the prevalence of obesity was lowest among children watching 1 or fewer hours of television a day, and highest among those watching 4 or more hours of television a day [Crespo et al. 2001].

Klesges RC et al. [1993] showed that television viewing affected the resting energy expenditure [metabolic rate] in children. This study sought to identify a metabolic mechanism that may explain the relationship between television viewing and obesity and to determine whether television viewing affected obese and normal-weight children differentially. Television viewing was found to acutely decrease resting energy expenditures in both normal-weight and obese children. There were no statistically significant differences in metabolic lowering between the two groups; however, the obese children experienced an average decrease of 265 kcal compared with 167 kcal for normal-weight children. It was also noted that in general, obese children watch more television per day than normal-weight children and would likely have lower metabolic rates over time compared with normal-weight children.

The Maltese 2007 Lifestyle Survey (Table 2) has confirmed that overall the young adult population are not particularly keen to perform regular physical exercise. Overall about half of the young adult population does not even attempt basic exercise in the form of a 30-minute walk a week. Only about 17.2% actually attend a gym or physical fitness club at least once a week [N.S.O., 2009].

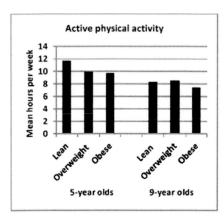 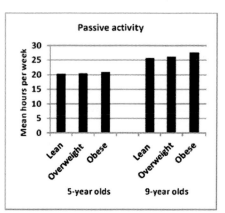

Figure 7. Physical activity reported in 5-year-old and 9-year-old children [after Scerri and Savona-Ventura, 2011].

This general trend to reduced physical activity was evident in Maltese children, particularly if adipose. Five and nine-year children report less mean active physical activity time than their leaner counterparts. Conversely mean passive activity time increased minimally with increasing adiposity particularly in the nine-year-old group (Figure 7). The differences were however not statistically significant [Scerri and Savona-Ventura, 2011].

TRANSGENERATIONAL DETERMINANTS

A number of studies have confirmed the adage that "obesity begets obesity" with the observation that obese parents often have children suffering from adiposity [Birch and Fisher, 1998]. A number of genetic determinants have been identified as contributory towards the development of adiposity insulin resistance and earlier susceptibility to develop T2DM. This gene polymorphism seems to predominantly express itself in adipose tissue to regulate lipid metabolism and thermogenesis. [Bouchard and Perusse, 1996; McCarthy and Zeggini, 2007]. An inter-relationship with inflammation has also been described [Shoelson et al. 2006; O'Rourke, 2009]. The reported data remains conflicting [Froguel and Velfo, 2002; Bouchard and Perusse, 1996]. In the Maltese population, a number of gene alleles representing metabolic syndrome genes, MODY genes and inflammatory response genes have been linked to Type 2 and gestational diabetes mellitus (Table 3)[Al-Ashtar, 2008; Abou-Hussein, 2009].

Table 3. Alleles contributing to T2DM and GDM in the Maltese population [after Al-Ashtar, 2008; Abou-Hussein, 2009]

Contributor alleles	Inflammatory alleles	IL-6 rs1800795 C/G
		TNDM rs4828037 C/T
		IL1RN BB/BC
		IL4 [B1B2]
		IL-6 -174 G/C
		MTHFR nt 677C/T
	Metabolic alleles	FTO rs9939609 A/T
		TCF7L2b rs12255372 G/T
		FABP2 codon 54 G/A
		UCP1 nt3826 A/G
		TCF7L2a IVS3 T/G
		Adrabβ2 nt46 A/G
	Inflammatory and Metabolic alleles	MIF -173 G/C
		Leptin nt -2549 C/A
Protective alleles	Metabolic alleles	SLC2A2 rs5393 A/C
		PAX4 rs2233578C/T
		UCP3 rs1800849 C/T
		IDE rs12356364 C/T
		CDKNN2A/2B rs10811661 C/T

The assessment of these alleles may help to develop a genetic susceptibility profile for individuals allowing for early timely intervention strategies to be developed [Abou-Hussein et al. 2011; Pace et al. 2012].

Three generational follow-up studies in the Maltese population have suggested that maternal obesity predisposes to macrosomia, particularly if associated with excessive weight gain during pregnancy [Savona-Ventura et al. 2008]. This increased mean birth weight noted in children of adiposed women in turn predisposes the child to future adult adiposity. Comparing adipose and lean 1st generation women has demonstrated an apparent link between adiposity in 1st generation women to higher mean birth weights in 2nd generation female children who in adulthood were more likely to become adipose. These in turn had 3rd generation infants of a higher birth weight. However, the link does not appear to be primarily genetic since the risks of high mean birth weights in the 3rd generation children was a correlate to their mother's adult BMI and not to the grandmother's BMI (Table 4) [Agius et al. in preparation].

year-old Maltese boys attending state schools [17.2 $\pm$ 3.2, n = 1018] was statistically [p = 0.001] higher than that of comparative children attending private schools [16.5 $\pm$ 2.0, n = 248]. No statistically significant difference was noted in the mean BMI of 6-year-old girls [state schools: 16.9 $\pm$ 2.9, n = 832 vs. private schools: 17.1 $\pm$ 3.1, n = 141: p = 0.44]. A similar relationship of higher mean BMI in boys, but not girls, attending state schools as compared to private schools persisted in the same cohort at 9 years of age [Farrugia Sant'Angelo and Grech, 2011]. Children attending private schools are assumed to belong to higher socio-economic groups than those attending state schools, and it is assumed that the observed tendency towards higher mean BMI in boys attending state schools reflect influences by parents and their social context of eating. In addition, the different school activities programmes are different between the schools. Different schools have different sports facilities and a survey carried out as part of the European Child Growth Surveillance Initiative in 2008 showed that the time spent in physical activity in higher in private schools as compared to state schools in Malta [Sammut, 2008 as cited in Farrugia Sant'Angelo and Grech, 2011]. It thus appears that whereas adiposity transgresses all social strata of the population, it is more prevalent in low socio-economic groups. Another study carried out in five and nine-year-old Maltese children using different indirect measures of socio-economic status – notably household size, single adult in household, and parental educational and occupation status – failed to show any statistical significant correlations [Scerri and Savona-Ventura, 2011].

Furthermore, there is accumulating evidence for the detrimental effects of over-controlling parental behaviour on children's ability to self-regulate energy intake. Parents are shown to influence children by child-feeding practices they implement from birth to adolescence, by the foods they make available at home, by direct modelling of eating behaviour, and by the way they engage with the children during meal times. Moreover, parents can influence their child's food preferences by adopting certain feeding strategies, such as the implementation of coercion, high levels of control, food rewards and bribery [Birch and Fisher, 1998]. Studies carried out to investigate the effects of parental control on the child's eating behaviour have had contradictory results. On the one hand, research has suggested that high levels of parental control may result in children developing maladaptive eating behaviour that may develop into overeating and obesity [Johnson and Birch, 1994]. On the other hand, Brown and Ogden [2004] report that high levels of parental control were associated with higher intakes of healthy snack foods. This contradiction may be explained by the type of control implemented by the parents. It is possible for a parent to control what their child eats by managing the environment. This is done by avoiding places which sell unhealthy foods and by only bringing healthy foods into the house. This form of control is called covert control since it is not apparent to the child. This control is also based on the theory that children model their behaviour to their parents and will thus adopt the same lifestyle choices as their parents [Brown and Ogden, 2004]. In contrast, overt control is the implementation of monitoring and restriction where the parents limit the child's intake of unhealthy foods in a way that can be perceived by the child [Ogden et al. 2006]. Research suggests that such parental practices may either be associated with disinhibition and overeating [Fisher and Birch, 1999], or alternatively may promote a predisposition towards eating an increased proportion of healthy snacks [Ogden et al. 2006]. The different results obtained by different workers may in part be influenced by the cultural perception of the parent-child relationships which vary from one community to another.

A three-generation study carried out in 2012 investigating the relationship between the young Maltese adult [18-26-year old] daughter's eating habits and the eating and parenting attitudes of the mother and grandmother suggested that women attitudes towards eating habits have changed significantly with a decline in healthy eating behaviour from mothers to daughters [Savona-Ventura, 2012]. There were further differences in body concern scores with the older generation showing greater concern than the younger ones. Attitudes towards maternal autonomy increased with increasing age with a corresponding reversal in attitudes towards daughter's autonomy (Table 5).

Table 5. Differences between three generations of women
[after Savona-Ventura, 2012]

	Daughter N = 50	Mother N = 50	Grandmother N = 50
Mean age [years]	21.3 + 2.7	51.4 + 4.7	78.5 + 6.6
Mean BMI [kg/m2]	24.8 + 4.2	28.0 + 6.0	27.7 + 4.6
Mean eating score *	0.46 + 1.02	1.23 + 1.14	1.09 + 0.98
Mother autonomy score	2.07 + 0.78	3.42 + 0.67	3.66 + 3.66
Daughter autonomy score	3.87 + 0.68	3.57 + 0.90	3.43 + 0.85
Body concern score	3.46 + 0.99	4.17 + 0.68	4.43 + 0.64
Projection score	3.38 + 0.44	3.30 + 0.33	2.93 + 0.48

* A minus five score reflects very unhealthy dietary habits behaviour; a plus 5 score very healthy habits. Same applies for other scores.

**Table 6. Influence of parenting attitudes towards control and autonomy
to daughter's eating patterns [* = statistically significant]**

	Daughter healthy eating	Daughter unhealthy eating
Mother's healthy eating	R = 0.27 *	R = -0.18
Mother's unhealthy eating	R = -0.29 *	R = 0.23
Grandmother's healthy eating	R = -0.09	R = 0.07
Grandmother's unhealthy eating	R = -0.11	R = 0.18
Daughter 's attitudes on control	R = 0.32 *	R = -0.29
Mother's attitudes on control [significant for healthy eating in covert and monitor type of control]	R = 0.26 *	R = -0.16
Grandmother's attitudes on control [significant for health eating only in restrictive type of control]	R = 0.12	R = -0.10
Daughter's attitudes to parenting style	R =-0.19	R = 0.17
Mother's attitudes toparental style [significant for unhealthy eating only in authoritative parental style]	R = -0.10	R = 0.09
Grandmother's attitudes to parental style [significant for healthy eating only in permissive parental style]	R = 0.37 *	R = 0.20
Daughter's attitude to autonomy	R = 0.23	R = -0.35 *
Mother's attitudes towards autonomy	R = -0.11	R = -0.14
Grandmother's attitude to autonomy	R = -0.01	R – 0.08

The study further confirmed that, in the Maltese family environment, the mother's eating behaviour did appear to reflect positively the daughter's eating behaviour. This was however tempered by attitudes towards parenting styles and control with high levels of parental control apparently contributing towards healthy eating in the young adults (Table 6).

CONCLUSION

Adiposity has become a major public health problem that needs to be urgently addressed with a multifaceted proactive approach using a multidisciplinary team. The adage that "prevention is better than cure" is very relevant to this problem. Medical child health providers in Malta feel that they are poorly equipped and experienced to address the problem of childhood obesity in their clinical practice. Perceived competencies in these practitioners were poorest for behavioural management, family therapy and parenting guidance emphasising the need for a multidisciplinary approach. Reported barriers to child obesity management included lack of patient motivation and parental involvement, and lack of support service [Aquilina et al. 2012]. Prevention of childhood adiposity, and consequently adult adiposity, should follow early identification of at risk individuals and timely intervention with healthy lifestyle patterns.

Studies have identified a number of features which increase the risks of childhood adiposity. Intervention should be instituted immediately on the identification of any risk factor (Table 7).

Table 7. Risk factors for childhood obesity

Antenatal	Infant	Childhood
Maternal obesity	Macrosomic or large-for-gestational age infant at birth	Rapid weight gain during childhood
Maternal diabetes mellitus [T1DM, T2DM, GDM]	Low birth weight [Small for gestational age or prematurity]	Elevated age-standardised BMI
Excessive maternal weight gain during pregnancy	Bottle feeding or early weaning	Poor attendance to school physical exercise activities
Low socio-economic status	Rapid weight gain during infanthood	

Adipose mothers-to-be should be encouraged to attend dedicated pre-conception care clinics to be assessed for the presence of impaired glucose tolerance and to receive tailored nutritional advice with or without pharmacological intervention. The nutritional advice should be further supplemented by realistic physical exercise programs. The aim of these lifestyle interventions should not only be pre-conception weight reduction, but also to introduce correct lifestyle patterns suitable for weight and metabolic control during pregnancy. In the Maltese population, it appears that, in order to reduce the risks of large-for-gestational age infants, maternal weight gain during pregnancy should be not more than 10 kg [Savona-Ventura et al. 2008].

During intrauterine life, determinants for eventual childhood adiposity include situations where the infant is chronically overfed. These situations include diabetes in the mother, maternal obesity and excessive weight gain during pregnancy. Women with these metabolic problems should have very careful antenatal follow-up with careful dietary advice and the advocacy of regular physical exercise to ensure that the foetus-in-utero is not exposed to an environment of over-nutrition. The role of pharmacological interventions such as the use of metformin during pregnancy in pre-pregnancy impaired glucose tolerance, gestational diabetes, and obesity needs to be evaluated.

Further risk factors can be identified at birth or through regular follow-up during childhood. Parents, particularly mothers, of high risk children should be encouraged to adopt healthy nutrition patterns for the whole family starting with breastfeeding for the infant. Covert parental control of dietary practices has been found to be the better means of influencing Maltese children. In addition, early involvement in sport activities may hopefully translate to a continuing pattern of regular physical exercise that helps counter the tendency towards adiposity. This lifestyle intervention advice should be continuously promoted by the child health care providers who should adopt a proactive policy for identifying early the development of childhood adiposity.

An effective intervention programme needs to be instituted on a nation-wide basis using multidisciplinary teams at every intervention point ensuring regular follow-up with repeated attempts at motivation and re-enforcement of healthy lifestyle intervention of both the child and the parents. This requires a serious commitment by government and public health officials to significantly invest to build up sufficient personnel resources.

REFERENCES

Abou-Hussein S. *Allele Scoring of Genetic Risk in Previous GDM*. MSc thesis, Faculty of Medicine and Surgery, University of Malta, 2009.

Abou-Hussein S, Savona-Ventura C, Grima S, Felice A. Genetic factors in risk assessment for the development of type 2 diabetes mellitus in a small case series. *International Journal of Risk and Safety in Medicine* 2011, 23:1-5

Agius EA, Cachia EA, Leniker HM. Average birth weight in Malta. St. Luke's Hospital Gazette 1966, 1[2]:77-79.

Agius R, Savona-Ventura C, Vassallo J. *Transgenerational metabolic determinants of fetal birth weight*. In preparation.

Alaimo K, Olson CM, Frongilo Jr EA. Low Income and Food Insufficiency in Relation to Overweight US Children: Is There a Paradox? *Archives of Pediatric and Adolescent Medicine* 2001, 155:1161-1167.

Al-Ashtar A. *Molecular SNPlotypes™ with Common Alleles Reflects Expression Profile in Diabetes Mellitus Type 2*. PhD thesis, Malta: University of Malta Medical School, 2008.

Aquilina S, Bedford H, Attard Montalto S. Attitudes and skills of Maltese paediatricians and trainees regarding childhood obesity. *Malta Medical Journal 2012*, 24[suppl.]:41.

Attard Montalto S. Breastfeeding Malta 2002. *Malta Medical Journal* 2002, 14[1]:37-41.

Barker DJ. In utero programming of chronic disease. *Clin. Sci.* [Lond] 1998; 95[2]:115 -128.

Birch CC, Fisher JO. Children, food, eating, dieting, parenting: Development of eating behaviour among children and adolescents. *Pediatrics* 1998; 101:539-549.

Bouchard C. Current understandings of the etiology of obesity: Genetic and non-genetic factors. *Am. J. Clin. Nutr.* 1991, 53:1561S-1565S.

Bouchard C, Perusse L. Current status of the human obesity gene map. *Obesity Res.* 1996, 4:81-90.

Brown R, Ogden, J. Children's eating attitudes and behaviour: a study of the modelling and control theories of parental influence. *Health Education Research* 2004, 19[3]:261-71.

Carvalhal MM, Padez MC, Moreira PA, Rosado VM. Overweight and obesity related to activities in Portuguese children 7 - 9 years. *European Journal of Public Health* 2007, 17:42-46.

Cassar C. Everyday life in Malta in the nineteenth and twentieth centuries. In: The British Colonial Experience 1800-1960: *The Impact on Maltese Society*. V. Mallia-Milanes ed., Malta: Mireva Publications, 1988, 91-126.

Crespos CJ, Smit E, Troiano RP, et al. Television watching, energy intake and obesity in S children. *Arch. Pediatr. Adolesc. Med.* 2001, 155:360-365.

D.H.I.R. The European Health Examination Survey – Pilot Study 2010. *Directorate for Health Information and Research*, Malta, 2012.

D.H.I.R. *National Obstetric Information System* – Annual Reports: 1995-2010. Department of Health Information and Research, Malta, 1999-2011.

Dietz WH. The obesity epidemic in young children. *BMJ* 2001, 323:1331-1335.

Ebbeling CB, Feldman HA, Osganian SK, et al. Effects of decreasing sugar-sweetened beverage consumption on body weight in adolescent: A randomized controlled pilot study. *Pediatrics 2006*, 117[3]:673-680.

Fagot-Campagna A, Pettit DJ, Engelgau M, et al. Type 2 diabtes among North American children and adolescents: an epidemiologic review and a public health perspective. *J. Pediatr.* 2000, 136:664-672.

Farrugia Sant'Angelo V, Grech V. Comparison of body mass index of a national cohort of Maltese children over a 3-year interval. *Malta Medical Journal* 2011, 23[1]:34-39.

Fisher JO, Birch LL. Restricting access to a palatable food affects children's behavioural response, food selection and intake. *American Journal of Clinical Nutrition* 1999, 69:1264-1272.

Formosa C, Savona-Ventura C, Mandy A. Cultural contributors to the development of diabetes mellitus in Malta. *International Journal of Diabetes and Metabolism* 2012, 20:25-29.

Froguel P, Velfo G. Genetic determinants of type 2 diabetes. *Recent Prog. Horm. Res.* 2002, 56:91-105.

Galea G, Agius Muscat H, Bellizzi M, Spiteri N, Vassallo Agius P. A National anthropometric study on children in Malta. Contribution to the Malta Case Study for the International Conference on Nutrition in Malta. Department of Health, Malta [summarised in: *Food and health in Malta - situation analysis and proposals for action.* D.O.H., Malta, 1993].

Galea J. *Report on the Health conditions of the Maltese Islands for the year 1956.* Department of Health, Malta, 1958.

Grech ES, Savona-Ventura C. *The Obstetric and Gynaecological Service in the Maltese Islands: 1987.* Department of Obstetrics and Gynaecology, Department of Health, Malta, 1988.

Guo SS, Chumlea WC. Tracking of body mass index in children in relation to overweight in adulthood. *Am. J. Clin. Nutr.* 1999, 70[s]:145s- 148s.

Janssen I, Kat-marzyk PT, Boyce WF, et al. Comparison of overweight and obesity prevalence in school-aged youth from 34 countries and their relationships with physical activity and dietary patterns. *The International Association for the Study of Obesity* 2005, 6:126- 132.

Johnson LS, Birch LL. Parents' and children's adiposity and eating style. *Pediatrics* 1994, 94:5.

Johnson-Taylor WL, Everhart JE. Modifiable environment and behavioural determinants of overweight among children and adolescents: report of a workshop. *Obesity* 2006, 14[6]:929-966.

Katona G, Aganovic I, Vuskan V, Skrabalo Z. *The National Diabetes Programme in Malta - Final report Phases I and II.* WHO: Geneva, 1983.

Klesges RC, Klesges CM, Eck LH, Shelton ML. A longitudinal analysis of accelerated weight gain in preschool children. *Pediatrics* 1995, 95:126-130.

Klesges RC, Shelton MS, Klesges CM. Effects of television on metabolic rate: Potential implications for childhood obesity. *Am. Acad. Pediatrics* 1993, 91[2]:281-286.

Lobstein T, Baur L, Uauy R. Obesity in children and young people: a crisis in public health. *Obes. Rev.* 2004, 5[1]:4-104.

McCarthy MI, Zeggini E. Genome-wide association scans for Type 2 diabetes: new insights into biology and therapy. *Trends in Pharmacological Sciences* 2007, 28[12]: 598-601.

Muller MJ, Mast M, Asbeck I, et al. Prevention of obesity – is it possible? *Obes. Rev.* 2001, 2[1]:15-28.

N.S.O. *Lifestyle Survey: 2007.* National Statistics Office, Malta, 2009.

N.S.O. *Demographic Review 2010.* National Statistics Office, Malta, 2011.

N.S.O. *Malta in Figures 2012.* National Statistics Office, Malta, 2012.

Nicklas TA, Elkasabany A, Srinivasan SR, Berenson G. Trends in nutrient intake of 10-year-old children over two decades [1973-1994]: the Bogalusa Heart Study. *American Journal of Epidemiology* 2001, 15:969-977.

Ogden J, Reynolds R, Smith, A. Expanding the concept of parental control: A role for overt and covert control in children's snaking behaviour? *Appetite* 2006, 47:100-106.

O'Rourke RW. Molecular Mechanisms of Obesity and Diabetes: at the intersection of weight regulation, inflammation, and glucose homeostasis. *World Journal of Surgery* 2009, 33[10]:2007-2013.

Pace NP, Felice AE, Vassallo J. Scoring genetic risk and biological/clinical endpoints in type 2 diabetes mellitus. *Malta Medical Journal* 2012, 24[suppl.]:12.

Pettit DJ, Baird HR, Alech KA, et al. Excessive obesity in offspring of Pima Indian women with diabetes during pregnancy. *NEJM* 1983, 308[5]:242-245.

Ravelli AC, Stein ZA, Susser MW. Obesity in young men after the famine expression in utero and early infancy. *NEJM* 1976, 295[7]:349-353.

Ravelli AC, Van-Der MJ, Osmond C et al. Obesity at the age of 50 years in men and women exposed to famine prenatally. *Am. J. Clin. Nutr.* 1999, 70[5]:811-816.

Savona-Ventura C. *The Thrifty Diet Phenotype – A Case for endogenous physiological teratogenesis.* In: Engels J.V. [ed.]: Birth Defects: New Research. Nova Science Publishers, USA, 2006, 183-200.

Savona-Ventura C, Chircop M. Birth weight influence on the subsequent development of gestational diabetes mellitus. *Acta Diabetologica* 2003, 40:101-104.

Savona-Ventura C, Grech ES. Infant feeding in Malta. *Journal of Psychosomatic Obstetrics and Gynaecology* 1990, 11:107-117.

Savona-Ventura C, Grima S, Vella K. Maternal BMI and antenatal weight gain as determinants of obstetric outcome. *International Journal of Diabetes and Metabolism* 2008, 16:51-53.

Savona-Ventura C, Schranz AG, Chircop M. Family History in the Aetiology of Gestational Diabetes Mellitus and Type 2 Diabetes. *Malta Medical Journal* 2003, 15[2]:25-27.

Savona-Ventura C, Scerri C. Child anthropomorphy in the mid-20th century. *Malta Medical Journal*, in press.

Savona-Ventura C, Zammit K, Vella S. Starvation and the development of the Metabolic Syndrome. *International Journal of Diabetes and Metabolism* 2007, 15:1-3.

Savona-Ventura S. *Changes in parental control and parenting styles across three generations and their impact on dietary habits in Malta.* Thesis: MSc in Health Psychology, University of Surrey, U.K., 2012.

Scerri C, Savona-Ventura C. Early metabolic imprinting as a determinant of childhood obesity. *International Journal of Diabetes Mellitus* 2010, 2:175-178.

Scerri C, Savona-Ventura C. Lifestyle risk factors for childhood obesity. *Childhood Obesity* 2011, 7[1]:25-29.

Shoelson SE, Lee J, Goldfine AB. Inflammation and insulin resistance. The *Journal of Clinical Investigation* 2006, 116[7]:1793-1801.

Sobal J, Stunkard AJ. *Socioeconomic status and obesity: A review of the literature. Psycholog. Bul.* 1989, 105:260-275.

Strauss RS, Knight J. Influence of home environment on the development o obesity in children. *Pediatrics* 1999, 103[6]:e85.

Taveras EM, Berkey CS, Rifas-Shiman SL, et al. Associations of consumption of fried food away from home with body mass index and diet quality in older children and adolescents. *Pediatrics* 2005, 116[4]:e518-e524.

Thompson OM, Ballew C, Resnicow K, et al. Food purchased away from home as a predictor of change in BMI z-score among girls. *International Journal of Obesity and Related Metabolic Disorders* 2004, 28:282-289.

von Kries R, Koletzko B, Sauerwald T, von Mutius E, Barnert D, Grunert V, et al. Breast feeding and obesity: cross sectional study. *BMJ* 1999, 319[7203]: 147-150.

Wang Y, Lobstein T. Worldwide trends in childhood overweight and obesity. *International Journal of Paediatric Obesity* 2006, 1:11-25.

Waterland RA, Garza C. Potential mechanisms of metabolic imprinting that leads to chronic disease. *Am. J. Clin. Nutr.* 1999, 69[2]:179-197.

W.H.O. 10 things you need to know about obesity. *WHO European Ministerial Conference on counter-acting obesity.* Istanbul, Turkey, World Health Organization, Copenhagen, 2006.

Young LR, Nestle M. The contribution of expanding portion sizes to the US obesity epidemic. *Am. J. Public Health* 2002, 92:246-249.

Zammit V, Zammit P, Savona-Ventura C, Buhagiar A, Grech V. Maltese national birth weight for gestational age centile values. *Malta Medical Journal* 2010, 22[2]:19-24.

In: Childhood Obesity   ISBN: 978-1-62618-874-7
Editor: Callum G. Jackson   © 2013 Nova Science Publishers, Inc.

Chapter 4

CHILDHOOD OBESITY

*Ibrahim Elbayoumy**

Ports and Borders Health Division Shaab, Kuwait

ABSTRACT

Obesity is getting to be a more prevailing disease all over the world. It is estimated that there are nearly 250 million obese and overweight persons in the world. In the last three decades childhood obesity also got prevalent as high as 18-30% in developed countries such as USA, Italy, Germany and England. Also in the developing countries, obesity is increasing, according to the data collected by WHO from 94 countries. The mean prevalence of obesity is 3.3% in these countries. In African and Asian countries under weight is 2.5-3.5 times more prevalent than obesity.

It is well known that the risk of developing hypertension insulin resistance and hyperinsulinemia are high in the obese persons. Obesity is also an independent risk factor in coronary heart disease; childhood obesity also has been shown to be having such negative effects on health, such as hypertension, abnormal glucose tolerance, x-syndrome and

* Medical Doctorate of Public Health, Preventive and Social medicine Dr P.H., Associate professor of Public Health, Preventive and Social medicine, Tanta faculty of medicine-Egypt, Consultant of Public Mealth Ministry of Health (MOH)-Kuwait, MBchB, MSc. (Public Health) Dr PH (Public Health) Dip. (Hosp Admin), Dip. (Nutr)-MSc. Diabetes Care and Education-Dundee Faculty of Medicine-Scotland-UK Address: Administration of Public Health, Ports& Borders Health Division P.O. box35180 Shaab, 36052 Kuwait. Mail to: I.Elbayoumy@Dundee.ac.uk and ielbayoumy03@Gmail.com.

cardiovascular disease. Development of obesity is affected by many factors such as genetic, family history, lack of physical activity, gender, income and nutritional habits of fatty meals consumption.

Obesity Causes

Weight gain occurs when the person eats more calories than body uses up. If the food you eat provides more calories than your body needs, the excess is converted to fat. Initially, fat cells increase in size. When they can no longer expand, they increase in number. If the person loses weight, the size of the fat cells decreases, but the number of cells does not.

Obesity, however, has many causes. The reasons for the imbalance between calorie intake and consumption vary by individual. Age, gender, genes, psychological makeup, and environmental factors all may contribute.

o   Genes: genes may play a role in efficiency of metabolism and storage and distribution of body fat.
o   Family lifestyle: Obesity tends to run in families. This is caused both by genes and by shared diet and lifestyle habits. If one of the parents is obese, you have a higher risk of being obese.
o   Emotions: Some people overeat because of depression, hopelessness, anger, boredom, and many other reasons that have nothing to do with hunger. This doesn't mean that overweight and obese people have more emotional problems than other people. It just means that their feelings influence their eating habits, causing them to overeat.
o   Environmental factors: The most important environmental factor is lifestyle. Your eating habits and activity level are partly learned from the people around you. Overeating and sedentary habits (inactivity) are the most important risk factors for obesity.
o   Sex: Men have more muscle than women, on average. Because muscle burns more calories than other types of tissue, men use more calories than women, even at rest. Thus, women are more likely than men to gain weight with the same calorie intake.
o   Age: People tend to lose muscle and gain fat as they age. Their metabolism also slows somewhat. Both of these lower their calorie requirements.
o   Pregnancy: Women tend to weigh an average of 4-6 pounds more after a pregnancy than they did before the pregnancy. This can compound with each pregnancy.

Certain medical conditions and medications can cause or promote obesity, although these are much less common causes of obesity than overeating and inactivity. Some examples of these are as follows:

o   Cushing syndrome
o   Depression
o   Certain medications (examples are steroids, antidepressants, birth control pills)
o   Prader-Willi syndrome
o   Polycystic ovarian syndrome

Obesity can be associated with other eating disorders, such as binge eating or bulimia.

The distribution of body fat also plays a role in determining your risk of obesity-related health problems. There are at least two different kinds of body fat. Studies conducted in Scandinavia have shown that excess body fat distributed around the waist ("apple"-shaped figure, intra-abdominal fat) carries more risk than fat distributed on the hips and thighs ("pear"-shaped figure, fat under the skin).

CHILDHOOD OBESITY

This term denotes an increase in total body fat. Body Mass Index (BMI) is a measure to determine childhood overweight and obesity. It is calculated using the adult's weight and height. BMI does not measure body fat directly, but it is a reasonable indicator of body fatness for most children and teens.

A child's weight status is determined using an age and sex-specific percentile for BMI rather than the BMI categories used for adults because children's body composition varies as their age varies between boys and girls. Overweight is defined as BMI at or above the 85th percentile and lower than the 95th percentile for children of the same age and sex using the National Center for Health Statistics reference population (1976-1980) [1].

Obesity is defined as BMI at or above 95th percentile for children of the same age and sex [2].

Obesity Causes

1.   Genetic syndromes associated with childhood obesity include the followings:

a. Prader–Willi syndrome i.e. obesity, narrow bifrontal diameter, small hands and feet and primary hypogonadism.
b. Laurence–Moon – Biel syndrome i.e. characterized by obesity, polydactyl and primary hypogonadism.
c. Pseudo hypo parathyroidism.
d. Cohen syndrome.
e. Down syndrome.
f. Turner syndrome.

It is reported that an ob gene is found on chromosome 7 and it is expressed only in the adipose tissue. It produces a protein called leptin which acts on the hypothalamus to reduce appetite. In the obese (ob ob) mouse, a mutation of the ob gene leads to production of protein which impairs the leptin feedback mechanism.

Also, impaired leptin receptor in the ventromedial nucleus of the hypothalamus resulting in increased release of transmitters such as neuropeptide Y normally stimulates feeding.

There is abundance of evidence that support genetic susceptibility as an important risk factor for obesity. Evidence from twin, adoption and family studies suggests that biological relative exhibit similarities in maintenance of body weight, and that heredity contributes five and 40 percent of the risk of obesity [2,3,4]. Other studies indicate that 50-70% of a person's BMI and the degree of adiposity (fatness) is determined by genetic influences and that there is 75 percent chance that a child will be overweight if both parents are obese, and 25-50 percent chance if just one parent is obese [5,6,7].

2. Hormonal disorders associated with childhood obesity include the following:
a. Growth hormone deficiency.
b. Growth hormone resistance.
c. Hypothyroidism.
d. Leptin deficiency or resistance to leptin action.
e. Glucocarticoid excess (Cushing syndrome).
f. Precocious puberty.
g. Polycystic ovary syndrome (PCOS).
h. Prolactin – secreting tumors.

3. Medications that may cause weight gain in children and adolescents include the following:
   a. Cortisol and other glucocorticoids.
   b. Megace: it is megestrol acetate, a synthetic derivative of naturally occurring steroid i.e. progesterone.
   c. Tricyclic antidepressants (TCAS).
   d. Monoamine oxidase inhibitors (MADIS), such as phenelzine.
   e. Oral contraceptives.
   f. Insulin (in excessive does)
   g. Thiazolidinediones.
   h. Risperidone.
   i. Clozapine.

Diagnosis of Obesity and Overweight

1. Comparison of the affected children with tables of ideal weight-height.
2. Calculation of body mass index (BMI) using the formula:

$$BMI = \frac{\text{Weight (kg)}}{\text{Height (m}^2)}$$

It is considered:

- Acceptable if 20-25 kg/m^2.
- Overweight of 27-30 kg/m^2.
- Obesity if it is over 30 kg/m^2.

3. Measurement of skinfold thickness over the middle of triceps muscles. Normally it is 20mm in men and 30 mm in women.
4. Dual–energy x-ray absorptiometry (DEXA) which is usually used to evaluate bone density provides the best assessment of total body fat.
5. Regional fat distribution can be determined:
   a. measuring the waist circumference. A waist circumference above 100 cm in men or 90 cm in women is associated with increased levels of triglycerides and reduced level of HDL-cholesterol.
   b. Calculating the ratio:
      Waist circumference
      Hip circumference

It Denotes

- Central (visceral) obesity if > 1.0 in men and > 0.9 in women.
- Peripheral (gluteofemoral) obesity if < 0.85 men and < 0.75 women.
    c. CT or MRI scanning of the abdomen. This provides an accurate estimation of visceral fat.

COMPLICATIONS OF OBESITY

1. Cardiovascular:
    a. Hypertension that is partly related to insulin resistance and hyperinsulinameia.
    b. Atherosclerosis due to increased levels of LDL and decreased level of HDL
    c. Arrhythmias and sudden death.

An increased risk of death from all causes and from coronary artery disease (CAD) has been consistently observed in males, but not in females, who had obesity during adolescence. In a follow-up of Harvard Growth Study, the risk of morbidity from CAD and atherosclerosis was increased among men and women who had been overweight (BMI> 75th percentile) as teenagers. The trend towards higher BMI values among ad descents in United States has been associated with increases in left ventricular mass, when compared to similar cohorts in earlier generations, further suggesting that obesity increases the long term risk for development of cardiac disease [8].

2. Endocrine:
    a. Non-insulin dependent diabetes mellitus (NIDDM).
    b. Insulin resistance leading to hyperinsulinaemia.
    c. Earlier menarche, greater frequency of irregular and anovulatory cycles and earlier menopause.
    d. Growth hormone is reduced but the insulin-like growth factor is normal (IGF).
    e. Triiodothyronine (T3) is increased by overfeeding and decreased with starvation.

Diabetes Mellitus

Epidemiological data, although limited, indicate that adolescent obesity is associated with increased morbidity and mortality in later life. Accordingly, the dramatic increase in the prevalence of type 2 diabetes mellitus among adolescent with obesity is likely to be accompanied by a host of diabetic-related complications in adulthood and reduction in the life span. Although obesity per se, is associated with heightened risk of morbidity related to abnormalities in glucose homeostatic, recent data indicate that the rate of increase in BMI during adolescence may also represent a significant risk factors for diabetes mellitus[8].

3. Pulmonary problems:
   Breathing problems, such as sleep apnoea can occur due to local fat accumulation in the tracheopharyngeal area [9]. Asthma also can occur in obese children [10].
4. Liver and gallbladder dysfunction:
   Evidence of liver dysfunction, with elevated plasma concentration of transaminases, is observed in 20% of children with obesity; the liver dysfunction most commonly reflects hepatic steatosis, but cirrhosis may develop in rare instances. Vitamin E supplements may be effective in reversing this so-called steatohepatitis, suggesting that the disorder reflect a state of vitamin E deficiency [11]. Cholethiasis is more common in adults with obesity other than in adult's normal weight. Although gallstones are usual in childhood, nearly one half of all cases of cholecystitis in adolescents are associated with obesity. Cholecystsitis may be even more common during rapid weight loss, particularly with very controlled-energy diets.
5. Orthopedic disorders:
   Numerous orthopedic disorders, including genu valgum, slipped capital femoral epiphysis, and tibia vara are observed more commonly in children with obesity.
   Excess weight in young children can cause bowing of the tibia and femurs; the resulting overgrowth of the proximal metaphysis is called Blount disease [12]. Also osteoarthritis and musculoskeletal discomfort [9].
6. Psychologic complications:
   Emotional and psychological sequelae are widespread. Anecdotal evidence suggests that depression and eating disorders are common in

children and adolescents referred to obesity clinics. Prejudice and discrimination against individuals with obesity are ubiquitous within US culture; even young children have been found to regard their peers who have obesity in negative ways. Social isolation, peer problems, and lower self-esteem are frequently observed.

7. Cancer:
   There is increased incidence of:
   Endometrial and postmenopausal breast cancer in women due to increased production of oestrogen from aromatization of circulating androstenedione in adipose tissue. Also increased possibility of incidence of colorectal and prostate cancer among men who had obesity as adolescents.

EPIDEMIOLOGICAL FEATURES OF CHILDHOOD OBESITY

Prevalence of Pediatric Obesity

The prevalence of overweight and obesity is increasing in both developed and developing countries, but at a very different speed and in different pattern [13]. Indeed, world Health Organization [14] where data obtained from the global database on obesity showed that 8.7% of adults were obese in 84 countries in 1999-2000. Odgen et al. (2006) [15] have reported a significant increase in the prevalence of overweight among children and adolescent (from 13.9% to 17.1%) and of obesity among adults (from 30.9% to 32.2%) during the 6-year period from 1999 to 2004 in the United States. In the US, the total cost of the overweight and obesity in 2000 by some estimates was 117$ billion with $ 61 billion direct and $ 56 billion indirect costs [16].

In gulf countries, Al Mousa and Parkash [17] have found that 4.7% of male and 6.7% of female preschool children (0 to 5 years) were obese. El-Bayoumy et al. 2009[18] have reported that the overall prevalence of overweight and obesity in adolescents in Kuwait aged (10-14 years) was 30.7 and 14.9% respectively.

In Saudi Arabia, Al Hazza 2007 [19] has reported that the prevalence of obesity among the school boys aged 6-14 years has increased seven times during 1988 and 2005 (from 3.4% to 24.5% respectively.

Must et al. [20] have reported that on excluding poor countries in the east Mediterranean region (e.g. Afghanistan, Djibouti, Mauritania, Somalia, Sudan and Yemen) the prevalence of overweight and obesity among schoolchildren aged 6-10 years was 12% and 25%, whereas among adolescents aged 11-18 years, it was 15% and 45%. By comparison, obesity has to been found to be 29% among Canadian children of similar age [21], 18% among American children [22], 26% among Italian children [23], 24% among New Zealand children [24] and 26% among Saudi adolescents aged 10 to 14 years [25].

FACTORS ASSOCIATED WITH OBESITY

1. Nutrition and Eating Habits:
Several studies have been published that attempt to link children's diets with incidence of obesity.

However, none have been able to show a causal link between diet and obesity [26, 27]. Two such studies include Bogalusa Heart Study and USDA Economic research service study.

- The Bogalusa heart study analyzed children eating patterns over two decades (1973-1994) using a series of seven cross-sectional survey given to 1584 ten year old children. The study discovered changes in children's eating patterns over this 20 year period including increased incidence of missed breakfasts, increased numbers of children eating dinner outside the home, and increased snacking. No causal associations were found between changes in meal patterns and overweight status [28].

- The USDA Economic research service study on fruit consumption indicated that higher fruit consumption is linked with lower BMI in both adults and children.
  A large cohort of 3064 children between the ages of 5 and 18 years were surveyed between 1994 and 1996 using the USDA's continuing survey of food intakes by individuals (CSFII). The study hypothesized that people who incorporate nutrient-dense, low-fat foods into their diets like those found in fruits and vegetables will have a healthy BMI. However, the study only found a weak correlation between body weight and vegetable consumption [29].

Economic improvement over the last 50% years in most of developing countries has resulted in greater affluence and to diets that are higher in fats especially saturated fat, cholesterol, and refined carbohydrates and low in polysaturated fatty acids and dietary fiber. This nutrition trend has also been accompanied with sedentary life style and increased level of stress. Consequently, the prevalence of obesity and other non-communicable diseases has risen steeply [30-31].

The nutrition transition can be noticed in all high income countries in the Arab Gulf countries where the people have high socioeconomic level. Several studies have reported the association of dietary patterns with obesity and central adiposity where western countries style has been present [31-32].

Hoppe et al. [33] have explored the potential link between intake as an infant and body size as well as body weight.

This Danish study of health term infants concluded that while protein intake (PI) in infancy as a predictor of future childhood weight and height, PI was not a predictor of obesity.

While authors noted a positive correlation between PI and height and body size at 9 months and 10 years of age, there was no correlation between PI and body fat at 10 years of age.

PI in infancy seems to stimulate early growth but these growth effects are not maintained through adolescence.

Armstrong and Reilly 2002 [34] have investigated the relationship between breast feeding and obesity in Scottish children. This large study of 32, 200 children demonstrated that the prevalence of obesity was lower in breast fed children as compared to formula fed children.

The data for this study (gathered from children 39-42 months of age) were adjusted to control for other variables such as socio-economic status, gender and birth weight. The authors also have noted that childhood obesity was also significantly and positively correlated with birth weight.

Dorosty et al. (2000) [35] have conducted a study for the association between adiposity rebound (AR) and dietary intake, parental BMI, Socio-economic status and childhood BMI. This longitudinal British study of 889 children followed from birth to 5 years concluded that while others reported evidence that AR, the time at which the BMI increases after it is lowest point in childhood is a critical period for the development of obesity, the authors could not substantiate the evidence.

In addition the study's authors concluded that there was no association between high protein intake or any other dietary variable and the timing of AR. The authors suggest that parental obesity was a better predictor of very early (at or above 43 months) or early (from 49 to 61 months) AR and childhood obesity as measured by BMI.

Although it is clear that the accumulation of excess calories and high caloric intake resulting from today's "obesogenic" environment shapes the children tendency to consume too much food, and too little exercise, three exists disagreement about the relative role of over-consumption and physical inactivity to the obesity epidemic in children. Considerable debate is ongoing in a diverse number of disciplines including economics, epidemiology and health services research. Some researchers have argued that the population trend in caloric intake has remained fairly constant and that changes in energy expenditure account for most of the increase in obesity prevalence [36-37]. Other researches have argued the opposite [38-39].

While there is no one definition of snacking, it is probably best to consider the content of snack foods and the increased eating frequency that snacking promotes as separate issues [40]. There is evidence from US that snacking prevalence i.e. occasions of snacking is increasing, The energy density of snack foods is increasing [41]. Snacks contribute to about 20-25% of total energy intake in countries like the US and UK [40]. However, there is a little evidence that a higher frequency of eating per se is a potential cause of obesity.

Cross-sectional studies tend to show a negative relationship or no relationship between meal frequency and BMI [42].

On the other hand of four cross-sectional studies with nationally representative population identified that, three studies have supported that energy intake as a primary determinant of childhood obesity [43-44], and one has supported that both energy intake and energy expenditure were the determinant of childhood obesity [45].

In the study of El-Bayoumy et al. (2009) [18] dietary intake obese and overweight Kuwaiti adolescents (10-14 years) was assessed by using 2 days 24 hours dietary recall and using food exchange lists where raw foods were converted into daily caloric intake. These food exchange lists were designed by the nutrition and food technology department – Faculty of Home economy – Menofiah University–Egypt. The study revealed that the majority of obese adolescents have reported a high intake of fast foods and soft drinks, frequent snacking, eating more than 3 meals per day and swallowing big pieces of food resulting in a high caloric intake per day.

2. Socio-Economic Status:

Among adults, a negative relationship between socioeconomic status (SES) (e.g., parental income, parental education, occupation) and being overweight or obese has been well established, however, the relationship appears weaker and less consistent in children [46-49]. The relationship between SES and obesity is complex. The patterns are more exaggerated in girls than boys and generally show that in low income countries, obesity is more prevalent in high SES individuals, and in affluent countries, it is more prevalent in low SES individuals [50]. The change in obesity prevalence patterns can be seen in some countries that have monitored obesity prevalence rates over a period of economic transition [51]. It seems that in developed countries, the relationship may be bi-directional (i.e. low SES promotes obesity and obesity promotes low SES) as well as both obesity and low SES being independently influenced by other common factors such as intelligence [50].

The mechanisms by which high SES in developed countries provides some protection against obesity have not been well characterized and are likely to be multiple, including behaviors such as restrained eating practices and increased levels of recreational activity, living in less obesogenic environment with greater opportunities for healthy eating and physical activity, and a greater capacity to manipulate their micro–environments to suit their needs. People living in low SES circumstances may be more at mercy of the increasingly obesogenic environment and end up talking the default choices on offer. Poorer neighborhoods tend to have fewer recreation amenities [52], be less safe and have higher concentrations of fast foods outlets [53].

A number of studies found that SES is negatively associated with children being overweight or obese [54]. It appears likely that the relationship between SES and obesity varies by race / ethnicity, such that the negative relationship is only apparent among white adolescent and is not apparent among Black or Mexican American adolescents in USA [55]. In other words, Black and Latino children from families with higher socio-economic status are no less likely to be overweight or obese than those in families with lower socio-economic status. Despite the more pronounced impact of SES among white children, T-they are substantially less likely to be overweight or obese than Black, Latino, or Native American children, who are disproportionately affected by obesity [56, 57].

In 1988, 12.5% of Black children and 21.8% of Latino children were overweight, while 12.3% of white children were overweight [58]. In 2003 regional survey in the Aberdeen area, American Indian boys' ages 5-17 years old had a prevalence of overweight at 22% and 18% for girls for the same age group [59].

Furthermore, the prevalence at which obesity has been increasing in children in the recent years has been even more pronounced and rapid among minority children: between 1986 and 1998, obesity prevalence among African American: and Hispanics has been increased 120%, as compared to 50% increase among non-Hispanic whites [60-61].

Findings from studies suggest that the effects of race/ethnicity and SES on the prevalence of childhood obesity cannot be individually determined because they are collinear. Therefore evidence is often inconsistent as a result of the difficulty of separating the overlapping factors [62]. Furthermore, the relationship among race/ ethnicity, SES, and childhood obesity may results from a number of underlying causes, including less healthy eating patterns (e.g. eating fewer fruits and vegetables, more saturated fats), engaging in less physical activity, more sedentary behavior, and cultural attitudes about weight [63].

Clearly these factors tend to co-occur and are likely to contribute jointly to differentials in increased risk of obesity in children.

Parental Influences

Numerous parental influences shape the eating habits of youth including. The choice of an infant feeding method, the foods they make available and accessible. The amount of time children are left unsupervised and their eating interactions with others in the social context. Several studies suggest that breast feeding offers a small but consistent protective effect against obesity in children [64]. This effect is most pronounced in early childhood. It has been hypothesized that exposure to complex sugars and fats contained in early childhood in bottle formula influence "obesogenic factors" in infants, which predispose them to weight gain later on life [65].

A recent study postulated that breast feeding may healthier eating habits because breastfed infants may eat until satiated, whereas bottle fed babies may be encouraged to eat until they have consumed all of the formula. Breast feeding also may expose babies to more variability in terms of nutrition and tastes since formula fed infants have experience with only single flavor, whereas breastfed infants are exposed to a variety of flavors from the maternal diet that are transmitted through the milk [66].

Research indicates that the perception of flavor in the mother's milk is one of human infant's earliest sensory experiences, and there is support for the idea that early experience with flavor has an effect on milk intake and the subsequent acceptance of a variety of food [67].

Studies suggest that parental food preferences directly influence and shape those of their children. In a study by Oliveria and colleagues, they reported that parents who ate diet high in saturated fats; they also had children who ate diet high in saturated fats [68]. It is suspected that this observation is not merely due to the foods parents feed their children, but rather due to the preferences children develop through exposure to foods that their parents refer early in their lives.

Birch and Fisher posit that exposure to fruits and vegetables and foods high in energy, sugar and fat may play an important role in establishing a hierarchy of food preferences and selection in kids [69]. Other studies have confirmed that availability and accessibility of fruits and vegetables was positively related to fruit and vegetables preferences and consumption by school [70]. Additionally, child-feeding practices that control what and how much children eat can also affect their food preferences, studies have determined that parents who attempt to encourage the consumption of foods may inadvertently cause children to dislike the foods. Whereas parents that attempt to limit foods may actually promote increased preference and consumption of limited foods in children [71-72].

Researchers also indicate that the social context in which a child is introduced to or has experiences with food is instrumental in shaping food preferences because the eating environment serves as a model for the developing child [73].

For many children, eating is a social event that often times occurs in the presence of parents, other adults, older siblings and peers. In these contexts, children observe the behaviors and of others around them.

These role models have been found to have an influential effect on future food selection, especially when the model is similar to the child, or perceived as being powerful as in the case of older peers [74-76].

Over the last three decades, there has been increase in the number of dual income families as more women have entered the workforce and there has been an increase in the number of women serving as the sole supporter for their families [77]. It has been hypothesized that increased rates and hours of parental employment maybe correlated with the weight increases in American children. Studies have demonstrated that children in single-parent families are more likely to be overweight or obese than children in two-parent families and that the rise in women working outside the home coincides with the rise in childhood weight problems [78-79].

Several potential mechanisms have been proposed to explain this phenomenon including the followings:

Constraints on parent's time potentially contribute to children overweight problems, as working parents probably rely more heavily than non-working parents on prepared, processed, and fast foods, which generally have high calories, high fat and low nutritional content.

- Children left unsupervised after school may make poor nutritional choices and engage in more sedentary activities.
- Child care providers may not offer as many opportunities for physical activity and may offer less nutritious food alternatives.
- Unsupervised children may spend a great deal of time indoors, perhaps due to safety concerns, watching TV or playing video games rather than engaging in more active outdoor pursuits (80).

3. Physical inactivity and sedentary behaviors:

Research indicates that a ↓ decrease in daily energy expenditure without a concomitant decrease in total energy consumption may be the underlying factor for the increase in childhood obesity. Physical activity trend data for children are limited, but cross sectional data indicates that one third adolescent are not getting recommended levels of moderate or vigorous activity, 10 percent are completely inactive, physical activity levels falls as adolescent age [81]. This situation may actually be worse than these data describe. Activity measured by physical activity monitors trends to be significantly lower than what is reported on surveys [82].

Watching television, using the computer and playing video games occupy a large percentage of children's leisure time, influencing their physical levels. It is estimated that children in the United States are spending 25% of their waking hours watching television and statistically, children who watch the most hours of television have the highest incidence of obesity [83-84].This trend is apparent not only because little energy is expended while viewing TV, but also because of the concurrent consumption of high-calorie snacks.

A recent examination of the department of Education's Early Childhood Longitudinal Survey (ECLS-K) found that a one-hour increase in physical education per week resulted in a 0.31 point drop (approximately 1.8%) in body mass index among overweight and at-risk first grade girls. There was a smaller decrease for boy. The study concluded that expanding physical education in kindergarten to at least five hours per week could reduce the percentage of girls classified as overweight from 9.8% to 5.6% [85].

Currently, schools are decreasing the amount of free play or physical activity that children receive during school hours. Only about one-third of elementary school children have daily physical education, and less than one-fifth have extracurricular activity programs at their schools. Daily enrollment in physical education classes among high school students ↓ decreased from 42% in 1991 to 25% in 1995, subsequently increasing slightly to 28% in 2003 [86].

Outside of school hours, only 39% of children ages 9-13 years participate in organized physical activity, although 77% engage in free-time physical activity [87]. In developing countries, data on population-based physical activity are very limited, for example a study on measuring physical activity in obese and non-obese 8-12 year school boys in Saudi Arabia using pedometer concluded that the prevalence of inactivity among boys was high (47%). However active boys showed significantly lower body fat percentage (P<0.01) and BMI (P<0.01) than inactive peers. Obese boys, on the other hand were significantly less active than non-obese boys (P<0.001) [88].

In Iran, Kelishadi et al. [89] have found that regular morning exercise was performed by school children at school, but there was no significant difference between girls and boys and between overweight or obese and other children for each sex.

In Kuwait, El Bayoumy et al. [18], physical fitness was assessed by modified Harvard step test. The majority of obese and overweight children i.e. more than 97% of them were physically inactive.

4. Television watching:

Several studies in Western countries have indicated that there is a positive association between the amounts of time spent watching television and obesity among children [90]. Increased television viewing time, playing video games, and using the internet have often cited as a contributing factor to the increased prevalence of sedentary behavior during leisure time, and therefore a decline in physical activity in Western countries [91].

In Saudi Arabia, it was found that obese preschool children (4-6 years) watched television significantly (p<0.001) longer than non obese (197.5 ± 89.3 and 150.0 ± 60.9 minutes per day respectively [92].

In Egypt, it was shown that 38% of non-obese preschool children aged 4-6 years watched television more than 2 hours per day, compared to 50% of obese children [93].

In Kuwait, sedentary life styles were encountered in obese and overweight children as playing video games and watching TV hours per day was 2.8 ± 1.9 in obese and overweight children compared with 2.7 ± 1.6 hours in normal weight children. Hours per day playing outdoors were 1.8 ± 1.5 hours in obese and overweight children compared with 2.1 ± 1.9 hours in normal weight children; sporting hours per week were reported as 4.8 ± 2.1 hours compared with 5.2 ± 2.9 hours in normal weight children [18].

CONCLUSION

The excess intake of calories above the daily expenditure of energy leads to weight gain and can eventually lead to obesity. The main components of this equation are energy intake (diet) and energy expenditure (physical activity, metabolic rate, etc.). The nutrition and physical activity habits of the population all over the world children have been changing over the past 40 years. Research shows some correlation of these changes to the increases in obesity levels in children. The physical environment, socio-economic status and race/ethnicity, family structure, genetics, and advertising may also influence diet and levels of physical activity among American youth.

Available research shows that there are a number of root causes of obesity in children. Selecting one or two main causes or essential factors is next to impossible given the current data, because the potential influences of obesity are multiple and intertwined. There are large gaps in knowledge, limiting the ability to pinpoint a particular cause and determine the most effective ways to combat childhood obesity. Another research gap stems from lack of a prospective longitudinal study that links dietary and other behavior patterns to development of obesity. Another complication of current data is that there is a need for more precise and reliable measures of dietary intake and activity levels, as individual recall of events and diet are not the most dependable sources for information.

When thinking about early prevention of obesity, it is essential that more is understood about how genetics is involved and how the genes are triggered or react to environmental changes and stimuli. Additionally, research is only beginning to explain how taste preferences develop, their biochemical underpinnings and how this information may be useful in curbing childhood weight gain.

Primary prevention is not an option for many children who are already overweight. Research on successful interventions for children who are overweight or at risk of becoming overweight is extremely important to effectively reduce childhood obesity in this country. Overall, research has just begun to scratch the surface in elucidating the causes of obesity in children. Filling in the knowledge gaps will take time, as implementing some of the study designs that will best illuminate the complex interactions are time consuming and costly. However the fundamentals are clear, to stay healthy, eat a balanced diet and devote adequate time to physical activity.

REFERENCES

[1]   Najjar MF, Bowland M. *Anthropometric Reference Data and Prevalence of Overweight-United States,1976-80DHHS publication no.(OHS)87-1688.*(Vital and health statistics;series11,no.238).Hyattsville, MD:US Department of Health and Human Services;1987.

[2]   Center for Disease Control. Factors Contributing to Obesity. Downloaded from: *www.cdc.gov/nccdphp/dnpa/obesity/contributing_factors.htm.* [Date accessed: December 12,2012]

[3]   Bouchard, C., Perusse, L. Genetic Aspects of Obesity. *Annals of the New York Academy of Sciences.* 699:26-35;1993.

[4]   Bouchard, C., Perusse, L., Rice, T., Rao, D. Genetics of Human Obesity. In: Bray, G.A, Bouchard, C. *Eds. Handbook of Obesity Etiology and Path physiology. 2nd Edition.* New York: Marcel Dekker 2003.

[5]   Skelton, J. Childhood Obesity: Overview. Downloaded from: *www.meadjohnson.com/professional/newsletters/0300app/0300a3.html.* [Date accessed: January 5,2013]

[6]   Jeffrey P. Koplan, Catharyn T. Liverman, and Vivica A. Kraak, Editors, Committee on Prevention of Obesity in Children and Youth. 2004. *Preventing Childhood Obesity: Health in the Balance.* Washington, DC: National Academies Press.

[7] In adults, Overweight is defined as a BMI (Body Mass Index) score of 25-29.9 and Obese is defined as a BMI score of 30 or greater. To calculate your BMI, go to: http://www.cdc.gov/nccdphp/dnpa/bmi/calc-bmi.htm [Date accessed: January 13,2013]

[8] Tirosh A,Shai I, Afek A, Dubnov-RAz,G, et al. Adolescent BMI trajectory and risk of diabetes versus coronary disease. N Eng J Med. Apr 7 2011:364 (14):1315-25.

[9] Han JC, Lawlor DA, Kimm SY. Childhood obesity. Lancet. May 15 2010:375(9727):1737-1748.

[10] Suther ER. Obesity and asthma. Immunol Allergy Clin North Am.2008:28(3):589-602, ix.

[11] Di Sario A, Candelaresi C, Ommenetti A, Benedetti A. Vitamin E in chronic liver diseases and liver fibrosis. Vitam Hom. 2007:76: 551-73.

[12] Taylor ED, Theim KR, Mirch MC, et al. Orthopedic complications of overweight in children and adolescents.Pediatrics.June2006; 1179(6): 2167-2174.

[13] World Health Organization(WHO).Obesity and managing the global epidemic. WHO technical reports series 894;1998, WHO, Geneva ,Switzweland.

[14] WorldHealth Organization(WHO). Nutrition data banks. Global data base on obesity and body mass index (BMI)in adults 2002.Available from http://www.who.int/db_bmi.htm. [Date accessed: January 20,2013]

[15] Odgen CL, Carroll MD, Curtin LR. McDowell MA. Prevalence of overweight and obesity in United States.1999-2004.JAMA 2006:295:1549-55.

[16] Wolf AM, Colditz GA. Current estimates of the economic cost of obesity in United States. Obes Res 1998;6:97-106.

[17] Al –Mousa Z, Parkash P. Prevalence of overweight and obesity among Kuwaiti children and adolescents. Bahrain Med Bull. 2002;22:123-127.

[18] El-Bayoumy I, Shady I, Lotfy H. Prevalence of obesity among adolescents (10-14 years) in Kuwait. Asia –Pacific Journal of Public Health. April 2009, volume 21,153-159.

[19] Al-Hazzaa HM. Prevalence and trends in obesity among school boys in central Saudi Arabia between 1988 and 2005.Saudi Medical Journal. 2007, volume 28,no.10,pp.1569-1574.

[20] Must A, Dallal GE, Dietz WH. Reference data for obesity :85th and 95th percentiles of body mass index(wt/ht^2) and triceps skin fold thickness. Am J Clin Nutr.1991:53:839-846.

[21] Young TK, Dean HJ, Flet B, Wood-Steiman P. Childhood obesity in a population at risk for type 2 diabetes mellitus .*J Pediatr*.200;136:366-369.

[22] Gathier BM, Hichner JM ,Qrnstien S. High prevalence of overweight children and adolescents in the practice of partner research network. *Arch Pediatr Adolesc Med*.200:154,625-628.

[23] Falorni A., Glamacci G., Bini V., Papi, F. Molinari D., De Giorgi G., et al. Fasting serum leptin level in the analysis of body mass index cut-off values: are they useful for overweight screening in children and adolescents? A school population – based survey in three provinces of central Italy. *Int. J.1998; Obes*. 22, 1197-12-8.

[24] Williams S. Body mass index reference curves derived from a New Zealand Birth. *Cohort. Nz. Med. J*.2000; 113, 308-311.

[25] Magobool G.M. Body mass index of Saudi children ages six to 16 years from the Eastern province. *Ann. Saudi. Med*.1994; 14, 495-498.

[26] Alexy U, et al. "Pattern of long-term fat intake and BMI during childhood and adolescence—results from the DONALD Study," *International Journal of Obesity* 2004; 28: 1203-9.

[27] Sugimori H, et al. "Analysis of factors that influence body mass index from ages 3 to 6 years—a study based on the Toyama Cohort Study," *Pediatrics International* 2004; 46: 302-10.

[28] Nicklas TA et al. "Children's meal patterns have changed over a 21-year period: the Bogalusa Heart Study *Journal of the American Dietetic Association* 2004 May: 104 (5):753-61.

[29] Lin, B-H and Morrison, RM. "Higher fruit consumption linked with lower Body Mass Index," USDA Economic Research Service *Food Review* Winter 2002; 25(3): 28-32.

[30] Galal O. Nutrition-related health patterns in Middle East. *Asia Pacific Journal of clinical Nutrition*.2003.vol.12,no.3,pp. 337-343.

[31] Ng SW, Zaghloul H I, Ali G, Harrison, Popkin. The prevalence and tends of overweight, obesity and nutrition-related non-communicable diseases in the Arabian Gulf States. *Obesity Overwei*. 2011. vol. 12, no.1, pp.1-13.

[32] Benjelloun S. *Nutrition transition in Morocco. Public Health Nutrition*. 2002. vol 5, no1A, pp.135-140.

[33] Hope C, Molgaard C, Thomsen B, Julul A, Michaelsen KF. Proten intake at 9 months of age is associated with body size but not with body fat in 10 years old. Danish children2004.American *Journal of Clinical Nutrition,* 79 (3); 494-502.

[34] Armstrong A, Reilly JJ. Breastfeeding and lowering the risk of childhood obesity. *The Lancet.*2003; 359(9352).

[35] Dorosty AR, Emmett PM, Cowin IS, Reilly JJ. Factors associated with early adiposity rebound. 2000. *Pediatrics*;105(5),1115.

[36] Heini AF, Weinstier RL. Divergent trends in obesity and fat intake patterns: the American paradox. *Am J Med* 1997; 102:259-264.

[37] Weinsier RL, Hunter GR, Heini AF, Goran MI, Shell SM. The etiology of obesity: relative contribution of metabolic factors, diet, and physical activity. *Am J Med* 1998;105:145-150.

[38] Bleich S, Cutler D, Murray C, Adams A. Why is the developed obese? *Annu Rev Public Health* 2008: 29:273-150.

[39] Hall KD, Guo J, Dore M, Chow CC. The progressive increase of food waste in America and its environmental impact. *PloS One* 2009; 4:e7940.

[40] Green SM, Burley VJ. The effects of snacking on energy intake and body weight. *Nutrition Bulletin BNF.*1996; 21:103-7.

[41] Zizza C, Seiga-Riz AM, Popkin BM. Significant increase in young adults: Snacking between 1977-1978 and 1994-1996 represents a cause of concern! *Preventive Medicine* 2001, 32(4):303-10.

[42] Drummond S, Crombie N, Kirk TA. Critique of the effects of snacking on body weight status. *European Journal of Clinical Nutrition* 1996; 50(12):779-83.

[43] Li S, Treuth MS, Wang Y. How active are American adolescents and have they become less active? *Obes Rev* 2010;11(12):847-862.

[44] Adams J. Trends in physical activity and inactivity amongst US 14-18 years old by gender, school grade and race,1993-2003:evidence from youth risk behavior survey. *BMC Public Health* 2006;6:57.

[45] Watkins DC, Murray L J, McCarron P, Boreham CA, Cran GW, Young et al. Ten years trends for fatness in Northern Irish adolescents: the Young Hearts Projects-repeat cross sectional study. *Int J Obes* (Land) 2005;29:579-585.

[46] Sobal, J. & Stunkard, A.J. Socioeconomic status and obesity: A review of the literature. *Psychological Bulletin, 1989;105*, 260-275.

[47] Strauss, R.S. & Knight, J. Influence of the home environment on the development of obesity in children. *Pediatrics, 1999; 101* (6).

[48] National Center for Health Statistics (1998). Health, United States with socioeconomic status and health chartbook. Hyattsville, MD.; Berkowitz, R.I. & Stunkard, A.J. (2002). Development of childhood

obesity. In Wadden, & Stunkard (ed). *Handbook of obesity treatment* (pp. 515-531).

[49] IOM (Institute of Medicine). 2005. *Preventing Childhood Obesity: Health in the Balance.* Washington, DC: National Academy Press.

[50] Stunkard AJ. Socioeconomic status and obesity. In: Cadwick DJ, Cardew G, eds. *The Origins and Consequences of Obesity.* Chichester: Wiley, 1996, 174–93.

[51] Monteiro CA, Conde WL, Popkin BM. Independent effects of income and education on the risk of obesity in the Brazilian adult population. *Journal of Nutrition* 2001; 131(3): 881S–6S.

[52] Subramania SV, Kawachi I, Kennedy BP. Does the state you live in make a difference? *Multilevel analysis of self-rated health in the US. Social Science & Medicine* 2001; 53(1):9–19.

[53] Reidpath DD, Burns C, Garrard J, Mahoney M, Townsend M. An ecological study of the relationship between socio economic status and obesogenic environments. *Health and Place* 2002; 8(2): 141–5.

[54] Sobal, J. & Stunkard, A.J. (1989); Strauss, R.S. & Knight, J(1989). Influence of the home environment on the development of obesity in children. *Pediatrics, 101* (6); National Center for Health Statistics (1998). Health, United States with socioeconomic status and health chartbook. Hyattsville, MD.; Berkowitz, R.I. & Stunkard, A.J. (2002). Development of childhood obesity. In Wadden, & Stunkard (ed). *Handbook of obesity treatment* (pp. 515-531).

[55] Troiano, R.P. & Flegal, K.M. Overweight children and adolescents: Description, epidemiology, and demographics. *Pediatrics, 1998;* 101 (3), 497-504.

[56] Crawford, Story, Wang, Ritchie & Sabry. Ethnic issues in the epidemiology of childhood obesity. *Pediatric Clinics of North America, 2001; 48* (4), 855-878.

[57] Strauss & Pollack. Epidemic increase in childhood overweight, 1986-1998. *Journal of the American Medical Association, 2001;* 286 (22), 2845-2848.

[58] Strauss RS, Pollack HA. Epidemic increase in childhood overweight, 1986–1998. *JAMA.*2001; 286:2845–2848. [PubMed]

[59] Zephier E, Himes JH, Story M. Prevalence of overweight and obesity in American Indian school children and adolescents in the Aberdeen area: A population study. *International Journal of Obesity,* 1999. 23, S28-S30.

[60] Alexander MA, Sherman JB, Clark L. Obesity in Mexican-American preschool children—a population group at risk. *Public Health Nurs.* 1991; 8:53–58. [PubMed]

[61] Sherry B, McDivitt J, Birch LL, et al. Attitudes, practices, and concerns about child feeding and child weight status among socioeconomically diverse white, Hispanic, and African-American mothers. *J Am Diet Assoc.* 2004; 104:215–221. [PubMed]

[62] Gordon-Larsen, P., Adair, L., & Popkin, B. The relationship of ethnicity, socioeconomic factors, and overweight in U.S. adolescents. *Obesity Research*, 2003 11(1), 121-12.

[63] Anderson, R. E., Crespo, C. J., & Bartless, S. J. Relationship of Physical Activity and Television Watching with Body Weight and Level of Fatness Among Children. *Journal of the American Medical Association,* 1998; 279(12), 938-942.

[64] Arenz S, Rucker R, and von Kries R. "Breast feeding and childhood obesity—a systematic review." *International Journal of Obesity* 2004; 28: 1247-1256.

[65] Yajnik, CS. "The lifecycle effects of nutrition and body size on adult adiposity, diabetes and cardiovascular disease." *Obesity Reviews* 2002; 3: 217-224.

[66] Bonuck, K et.al. "Is late bottle-weaning associated with overweight in young children? Analysis of NHANES III data. *Clinical Pediatrics (Philadelphia)* Jul.-Aug. 2004; 43(6): 535-40.

[67] Sullivan, S., Birch, L. Infant dietary experience and acceptance of solid foods. *Pediatrics.*1993,93:271-277.

[68] Oliveria, S. et al. Parent-child relationships in nutrient intake: the Framingham children's study. *American Journal of Clinical Nutrition.*1992, 56:593-598.

[69] Birch, L., Fisher, J. Development of eating behaviors among children and adolescents. *Pediatrics.*1998, 101:539-549.

[70] Hearn, M., Baranowski, T., and Baranowski, J. et al. Environmental influences on dietary behavior among children: Availability and accessibility of fruits and vegetables enable consumption. *Journal of Health Education.* 1998.

[71] Fisher, J., Birch, L. 3-5 Year-old children's fat preferences in consumption are related to parental adiposity. *Journal of the American Dietetic Assn*, 1995, 95:759-764.

[72] Center for Disease Control. Factors Contributing to Obesity. Downloaded from: *www.cdc.gov/nccdphp/dnpa/obesity/contributing_ factors.htm.* Accessed: Feb 18 ,2013.

[73] US Market for Kids Foods and Beverages, 2003. Kids' Lifestyles—US [Online] Downloaded from: *http://www.marketresearch.com/research index/849192.html#pagetop.* Accessed: Feb 20, 2013

[74] Birch, LL. Effects of peer models' food choices and eating behaviors on preschooler's food preferences. *Child Development.*1980 51: 489-496.

[75] Birch, LL. The relationship between children's food preferences and those of their parents. *Journal of Nutrition Education.*1980 12:14-18.

[76] Duncker, K. Experimental modification of children's food preferences through social suggestion. *Journal of Abnormal Social Psychology* 1983.33:490-507.

[77] Sado, S., Bayer, A. The Changing American Family. Downloaded from the Population Resource center website *http://www.prcdc.org/summaries /family/family.html.* Accessed Feb 2013.

[78] United States Census Bureau. 2000. *Statistical Abstract of the United States 2000.* Washington, DC: Government Printing Office.

[79] Jeffrey P. Koplan, Catharyn T. Liverman, and Vivica A. Kraak, Editors, Committee on Prevention of Obesity in Children and Youth. 2004. *Preventing Childhood Obesity: Health in the Balance.* Washington, DC: National Academies Press.

[80] Anderson, P., Butcher, K., and Levine, P. Maternal Employment and Overweight Children. *Journal of Health Economics,2003, 22,* 477-504.

[81] IOM, *Preventing Childhood Obesity: Life in the Balance,* 2004.

[82] Pate RR, Reedson PS, Sallis JF, Tayor WC, Sirard J, Trost SG, Dowda M. Compliance with physical activity guidelines: prevalence in a population of children and youth. *Annals of Epidemiology.*2002, 12 (5), 303-308.

[83] Robinson, T. N. Television viewing and childhood obesity. *Pediatric clinics of North America,* 2001, *48*(4), 1017-1025.

[84] CDC.Physical Activity Levels Among Children Aged 9-13 Years -- United States. *MMWR, 2003, 52*(33), 785-788.

[85] Ashlesha Datar, Roland Sturm. Physical Education in Elementary School and Body Mass Index: Evidence from the Early Childhood Longitudinal Study. *American Journal of Public Health.* 2004; 94 (9): 1501-1506.

[86] YRBSS Fact Sheet: Physical Activity. Found at: *http://www.cdc.gov/ HealthyYouth/yrbs/pdfs/trends-pa.pdf*

[87] Aaron DJ, Storti KL, Robertson RJ, Kriska AM, LaPorte RE. Longitudinal study of the number and choice of leisure time physical activities from mid to late adolescence: implications for school curricula and community recreation programs. *Arch Pediatr Adolesc Med.* 2002; 156(11):1075–80.

[88] Al –Hazza HM. Pedometer –determined physical activity among obese and non-obese 8-12 years old in Saudi school boys. *Journal of Physiological Anthropology*.2007; vol26, no.4, pp.459-465.

[89] Kelishai R, Hashemi Pour M, Sarraf-Zadegan et al. Obesity and associated modifiable environmental factors in Iranian adolescents: Isfahan Health Heart program-heart health promotion from childhood. *Pediatrics International* 2003, Vl.45, no.4, pp.435-442.

[90] Caroli M, Argentier L, Cardone M,, Masi A. Role of television in childhood obesity prevention. *International Journal of Obesity.* 2004,Vol.28, no.3, pp.S104-S108.

[91] Strauss & Pollack. Epidemic increase in childhood overweight, 1986-1998. *Journal of the American Medical Association, 2001;* 286 (22), 2845-2848.

[92] Al Hazza HM, Al Rasheedi AA. Adiopsity and physical activity levels among preschool children in Jeddah, Saudi Arabia. *Saudi Medical Journal.* 2007; vol.28, no.5, pp.766-773.

[93] Farahat TM, Mechael AA, Abu-Salem M. Prevalence of obesity among preschool children in Menofia-Egypt. *Arab Journal of Food and Nutrition 2006*, vol.7, no.15, pp.14-27.

In: Childhood Obesity   ISBN: 978-1-62618-874-7
Editor: Callum G. Jackson   © 2013 Nova Science Publishers, Inc.

Chapter 5

OBESITY AND MENTAL HEALTH IN THE YOUNG: A TWO-WAY STREET?

Valsamma Eapen[1] and Mukesh Prabhuswamy[2,]*

[1]Child and Adolescent Psychiatry, UNSW,
Academic Unit of Child Psychiatry South West Sydney (AUCS),
ICAMHS, Sydney South West Area Health
Service, Liverpool, NSW, Australia
[2]School of Medicine University of Western Sydney and
University of New South Wales, Gna Ka Lun Adolescent Mental
Health unit and ICAMHS South Western Sydney Local Health District
Campbelltown Hospital, Therry Road, Campbelltown,
NSW, Australia

ABSTRACT

In the last decade or so there has been an increasing awareness of the association between weight changes, mental health and psychotropic medications. The relationship is rather complex with changes in weight occurring as part of many psychiatric conditions including depression, eating disorders, ADHD, anxiety disorders and also just as part of stressful periods for an individual. The relationship gets more complex with medications especially Second Generation Antipsychotics (SGAs) used in the treatment of psychoses. There is a clear association with the

---

* Corresponding author.

use of medications, weight gain and medical morbidity. A big need of the hour is to look at pragmatic and informed approaches to intervention in these situations when weight gain becomes a commonly encountered accompaniment of psychiatric treatment. A preventive and early intervention focus is critical in the comprehensive management to avoid physical co-morbidity. This clinical review attempts to address some of these issues with a specific focus on metabolic syndrome.

Keywords: Psychiatric conditions, psychotropic medications, antipsychotics, psychoses, weight gain, medical morbidity, early intervention, metabolic syndrome

INTER-RELATIONSHIP BETWEEN MENTAL HEALTH AND OBESITY

Childhood obesity has been on the rise in the last two decades and has become a public health crisis in the 21st century. Though not the ideal parameter especially for the very young, Body Mass Index (BMI) is a good proxy measure for epidemiological studies of obesity. For the Western population a consensus committee (Spear et al. 2007) defined overweight as a BMI percentile between the 85-94% for age, obese as a BMI $\geq$ 95% for age, and severe obesity as a BMI percentile at 99% for age which corresponds to a BMI of 30-31 kg/m^2 for a 10-12 year old and a BMI of 34 for 14-16 year olds.

Studies indicate that 20% of school-age children in European countries and 30% in North America are overweight or obese (and 5 and 15 % meet criteria for obesity respectively) (Wang and Lim, 2012). The rates of obesity and being overweight have dramatically risen in developing countries as well (Eapen et al. 2010), particularly in the wealthy urban population (IOTF, 2007).

Childhood obesity has serious short and long-term consequences with significant long-term effects on mortality and morbidity (Dietz, 1998; Must & Strauss, 1999). Overweight and obese children are likely to maintain their status into adulthood and are at higher risks for developing chronic diseases such as hypertension, dyslipidaemia, type 2 diabetes, heart disease, stroke, gallbladder disease, osteoarthritis, sleep apnoea and respiratory problems, and certain cancers (WHO, 2010). The prevalence of type 2 diabetes has also been increasing among young people in many countries during recent years, largely due to obesity. Moreover, the obesity epidemic also has many economic consequences.

Many psychiatric disorders start during childhood and adolescence with approximately 22% of Adolescents in the US estimated to meet lifetime criteria for a mental disorder (Merikangas et al. 2010) and this rate is comparable to other parts of the world. Mental health and excessive body weight has a bidirectional relationship (Eapen and John 2011). There is evidence that the rates of mental health problems are more in children and adolescents who are overweight and obese. Further, obesity and being overweight has specific association with disordered eating behaviours, conditions such as ADHD, Depression, and also specifically with Antipsychotic treatment.

Disordered or Loss of Control eating (eating objectively large amounts with a sense of loss of control) has been found in up to 10% of children and adolescents in community samples (Wolkoff et al. 2011). This behaviour has been found to be associated with disordered cognitions about eating and body image (Hilbert et al. 2009) and is considered as a precursor of syndromal eating disorders and also weight gain and obesity. It has been found that mothers and children possibly share disordered eating patterns and this could explain the interpersonal causation of weight gain and obesity (Elliott et al. 2010). Youngsters with disordered eating have been observed to have higher ratings of anxiety, depression, negative moods and body dissatisfaction (Kalarchian and Marcus, 2012). Similarly, the rate of obesity has been found to be higher in children and adolescents with untreated ADHD and this population is more likely to report anxiety or depression as noted in a representative US and German sample (Waring and Lapane., 2008; Erhart et al. 2012). Further, a correlation between impulsivity, inattention and being overweight has also been reported.

MOOD AND OBESITY: CAUSE OR EFFECT?

The relationship between mood and obesity is bi-directional and the association cannot be fully explained by poor life style related risk factors as it persists even after controlling for these factors. Paediatric data indicate that girls are more vulnerable to comorbid mood and eating problems (Kendler et al. 1996). In this regard it is noteworthy that overweight and obesity in childhood tracks into adulthood with significant impact on both physical and psychological health. Those with major depressive disorder have been shown to have increased risk of developing overweight and obesity and vice versa. Moreover, studies examining the phenomenology, comorbidity, family history, biological, and hormonal factors in mood disorders and obesity show that both conditions share many similarities. Given the role of unhealthy lifestyle (poor dietary choices, lack of exercise) in the etiology, overlapping pathophysiological mechanisms in the course, as well as the negative impact of poor compliance to therapeutic programs in the prognosis, it is important to consider psychosocial issues in the management of obesity and Metabolic Syndrome (MS). It is to be noted that psychosocial factors and mood symptoms may play an important role in the chain of events that lead to MS and these factors would deserve special consideration in the comprehensive management of these patients.

MENTAL HEALTH DISORDERS AND METABOLIC SYNDROME

What Is Metabolic Syndrome?

Metabolic Syndrome (MS) is defined as a clustering of abnormalities such as hypertension, impaired glucose (insulin resistance; glucose intolerance or type 2 diabetes) and lipid metabolism (low HDL; hypertriglyceridemia) as well as central obesity (high waist-to-hip ratio) as defined by the National Cholesterol Education Program Adult Treatment Panel III (ATP III) (2001).

Antipsychotics and Weight Gain

There has been an exponential increase in prescribing SGAs since they became available. In outpatient settings, Olfson et al. noted a 6-fold increase between 1993 and 2002. However, growing evidence suggests an association between SGAs and a worsening in metabolic parameters. There is a big concern about psychotropic-induced weight gain, obesity, hyperlipidemia, impaired glucose tolerance, and diabetes mellitus with far reaching adverse consequences in the young population (Eapen V, Curtis J, Shiers D 2012).

A review of the child and adolescent literature (Briles et al. 2012), indicates that apart from some differences between specific medications, SGAs are more associated with weight gain and metabolic abnormalities. The worst offender was noted to be Olanzapine with an average weight gain of 6-8 kg over a 10-week period. This was comparable and followed by Risperidone,

Quetiapine and Clozapine. The least propensity for weight gain seems to be with Ziprasidone and Aripiprazole. The authors commented that no studies had addressed the question of whether the observed weight gain is a direct result of the growing trend in obesity in society, or the medications themselves, or a combination of the two and believed these to be important areas for further exploration.

Mediators in the Pathogenesis of MS

While there is no single causative factor for MS (Grundy et al. 2005), several psychosocial factors including personality characteristics and stressful life events have been implicated as predictors of metabolic abnormalities as well as cardiovascular and related morbidity and mortality (Lakka et al. 2002).

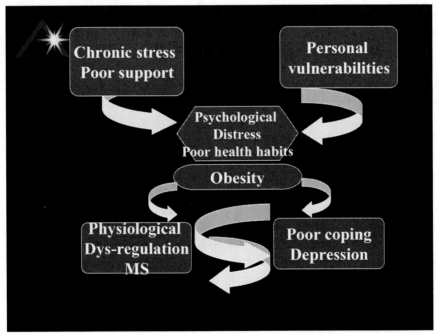

Reversing the trend: What can be done to prevent the occurrence and progression of weight gain and related complications in the mentally ill young people?

Figure 1. Inter-relationship between individual, life style and psychological factors in causing MS and depression.

Several pathophysiological mechanisms are under play with depressive symptoms and intense and frequent feelings of anger, as well as marital dissatisfaction, divorce, and widowhood being shown to predict increasing risk for MS. A subsequent study by the same investigators (Räikkönen et al. 2007) examined whether psychosocial factors that are related to cardiovascular disease and type 2 diabetes predict prospectively the risk for MS. In a cohort of women who did not have MS at the baseline, they found that the risk for MS varied from 1.21- to 2.12-fold for more severe depressive symptoms or very stressful life event(s). Thus, subjects with MS are at increased risk of developing mood symptoms and vice versa with common mediators such as genetic, environmental and life style factors suggested for depression, abdominal obesity and glucose levels. Stress and psychological distress mediated through disordered eating and obesity can lead to both MS and depression (Figure 1).

Interventions

For a detailed overview on interventions in Paediatric obesity, readers are referred to the paper by Scheimann (2012). The paper spells out that the goal of management is promotion of a healthy lifestyle to improve energy balance through improved diet and physical activity. It is reported that positive results are obtainable with low fat and low glycaemic index diets rather that dietary restriction which can be quite difficult to implement in young people with a mental illness. Engaging in regular physical activity through participation in a gym or an exercise regime is not always feasible in this population. Hence targeting sedentary lifestyle may be a better strategy and involving kids in free play may be more effective. The review also mentions albeit with a word of caution about the likely utility of medications such as stimulants, appetite suppressants, Rimonabant and Orlistat and the role for bariatric surgery in those adolescents who develop morbid obesity. However none of these have been specifically used in atypical antipsychotic-induced weight gain.

Metabolic assessments that will need to be carried out in young patients on SGAs include triglycerides, total cholesterol, high density lipoprotein (HDL) cholesterol, blood glucose, and haemoglobin A1c and insulin sensitivity. In this regard, it is important to screen patients for being " at risk for adverse health outcome " according to Correll and Carlson (2006) criteria and for features of metabolic syndrome as per the National Cholesterol Education Program's Adult Treatment Panel III Criteria modified by Cook for use in young people (Cook et al. 2003). The assessment in these cases should include weight and BMI; waist circumference; blood pressure; lipid levels; and glucose levels. According to the American Diabetes Association – American Psychiatric Association (ADA–APA) Consensus Guidelines (2004), weight should be assessed at four, eight, and 12 weeks after initiating or changing an antipsychotic agent, and quarterly thereafter. Fasting plasma glucose levels, lipid profile, and blood pressure should be assessed every three months on initiation of antipsychotic therapy, and sooner in persons who are at high risk at baseline. Compared with a fasting glucose test, a post-load oral glucose tolerance test is an earlier indicator of failing glucose control.

Other important and potentially modifiable risk factors may also warrant consideration, including elevated levels of low-density lipoprotein (LDL) cholesterol, family history of premature coronary heart disease, diet, smoking, alcohol and substance use, and exercise or lack of activity either with or without weight changes.

There is some evidence that Waist Circumference measurement is a simple and sensitive screening tool for determining the risk for MS (Panagiotopoulos et al. 2012). More data is needed to establish if this alone is sensitive enough and whether it can be used in the community by general practitioners while following-up SGA treated children and adolescents.

There is emerging literature in adults which suggests that non-pharmacological management is effective in reducing the weight gain induced by SGAs. Considering that weight gain can occur quite rapidly in children and adolescents, a primary prevention approach is critical as is the case in many lifestyle related disorders. Once the weight gain sets in, it quickly impacts on the young person's body image and self-esteem which can be detrimental to the psychological improvement. Furthermore, the medical morbidity can have devastating effects as already discussed.

Health promotion as well as intensive lifestyle and behavioral programs (Alvarez-Jimenez et al. 2008b; Brar et al. 2005; Curtis et al. 2011; Curtis et al. 2012; Kwon et al. 2006) should be made available for all patients through community clinics at each visit, routinely including youth-friendly intervention strategies incorporating dietary counselling, exercise programs and information on healthy living to prevent weight gain occurring, and to assist those who have gained excess weight to lose it and remain at healthy levels (Eapen, 2012; Eapen et al 2012). It is important to pay attention to co-morbid substance use especially nicotine use as this can aggravate the risks associated with the metabolic syndrome.

The key components of the preventive programme involving a multi-disciplinary team should include (Eapen et al. 2012),

1. Dietary counselling and Lifestyle modification with focus on eating habits, physical activity etc.
2. Educational strategies focusing on risk and resilience factors.
3. Individual therapy to address mood and psychological issues and to improve motivation to enact life style changes
4. Family support and interventions.

The authors have suggested that sociodemographic factors, personal and clinical factors including co-morbidities have to be addressed concurrently while using the above components.

In conclusion, the metabolic effects of SGAs in children and adolescents can have potentially devastating consequences. Of particular concern are the cardiovascular outcomes. A preventive approach that is very early in the course after initiation of treatment needs to be followed up by specialist mental health service providers in conjunction with support from GPs in the community. This is likely to be the most pragmatic approach in preventing the long-term physical morbidity in this vulnerable population.

REFERENCES

ADA–APA (2004) Consensus development conference on antipsychotic drugs and obesity and diabetes. *Journal of Clinical Psychiatry* 65:267–272. Eapen V (2012). Metabolic monitoring for patients on antipsychotic medication: are we failing to provide reasonable standard of physical healthcare? *Evid. Based Nurs.* 2012 Jul; 15(3):97-8.

Adult Treatment Panel III (2001). Executive summary of the Third Report of the National Cholesterol Education Program (NCEP) Expert Panel on Detection, Evaluation, Treatment of High Blood Cholesterol in Adults. *JAMA*, 285, 2486–2497.

Bayoumi RA, Al-Yahyaee SA, Albarwani SA, Rizvi SG, Al-Hadabi S, Al-Ubaidi FF, Al-Hinai AT, Al-Kindi MN, Adnan HT, Al-Barwany HS, Comuzzie AG, Cai G, Lopez-Alvarenga JC, Hassan MO (2007). Heritability of determinants of the metabolic syndrome *Obesity*, 15, 551-556.

Briles JJ, Rosenberg DR, Brooks BA, Roberts MW, Diwadkar VA (2012). Review of the safety of second-generation antipsychotics: are they really "atypically" safe for youth and adults? *Prim. Care Companion CNS Disord.* 14(3). pii: PCC.11r01298. doi: 10.4088/ PCC.11r01298. Epub 2012 Jun 7.

Brunner EJ, Hemnigway H, Walker BR, Page M, Clarke P, Juneja M, Shipley MJ, Kumari M, Andrew R, Seckl JR, Papadopoulos A, Checkley S, Rumley A, Lowe GDO, Stansfeld SA, Marmot MG (2002). Adrenocortical, autonomic and inflammatory causes of the metabolic syndrome. *Circulation*, 106, 2659–2665.

Cook S, Weitzman M, Auinger P, Nguyen M, Dietz WH (2003) Prevalence of a metabolic syndrome phenotype in adolescents: findings from the Third National Health and Nutrition Examination survey, 1988-1994. *Arch. Pediatr. Adolesc. Med.* 157: 821-827.

Correll CU, Carlson HE (2006). Endocrine and metabolic adverse effects of pychotropic medications in children and adolescents. *J. Am. Acad. Child and Adolesc. Psychiatry* 45:771-791.

Dietz WH (1998). Health consequences of obesity in youth: childhood predictors of adult disease. *Pediatrics.* 101(3 Pt 2):518-25.

Eapen V, John G (2011). Weight gain and metabolic syndrome among young patients on antipsychotic medication: what do we know and where do we go? *Australas Psychiatry.* 19(3):232-5.

Eapen V, Mabrouk A, Yousef S (2010). Metabolic Syndrome among the young obese in the United Arab Emirates. *Journal of Tropical Pediatrics*, 55: 46-48.

Eapen V, Shiers D, Curtis J (2012). Bridging the gap from evidence to policy and practice: Reducing the progression to metabolic syndrome for children and adolescents on antipsychotic medication. *Aust. N. Z. J. Psychiatry* Oct 9. [Epub ahead of print].

Elliott, C. A., Tanofsky-Kraff, M., Shomaker, L. B., Columbo, K. M., Wolkoff, L. E., Ranzenhofer, L. M.,Yanovski, J. A (2010). An examination of the interpersonal model of loss of control eating in children and adolescents. *Behaviour Research and Therapy*, 48, 424– 428.

Erhart, M., Herpertz-Dahlmann, B., Wille, N., Sawitzky-Rose, B., Holling, H. & Ravens-Sieberer, U (2012). Examining the relationship between attention-defi cit/hyperactivity disorder and overweight in children and adolescents. *European Child & Adolescent Psychiatry*, 2, 39 – 49.

Grundy SM, Cleeman JI, Daniels SR, Donato KA, Eckel RH, Franklin BA, Gordon DJ, Krauss RM, Savage PJ, Smith SC Jr, Spertus JA, Costa F

(2005). Diagnosis and management of the metabolic syndrome: an American Heart Association/National Heart, Lung, and Blood Institute Scientific Statement. *Circulation*, 112, 2735–2752.

Hilbert, A., Rief, W., Tuschen-Caffi er, B., de Zwaan, M. & Czaja, J (2009). Loss of control eating and psychological maintenance in children: An ecological momentary assessment study. *Behaviour Research and Therapy*, 47, 26 – 33.

IOTF (2007). Worldwide prevalence of obesity. *International Obesity Task Force*. http://www.iotf.org.

Kalarchian MA, Marcus MD (2012). Psychiatric comorbidity of childhood obesity. *Int. Rev. Psychiatry*. 24(3):241-6.

Kendler, K. S., Eaves, L. J., Walters, E. E., Neale, M. C., Heath, A. C. & Kessler, R. C (1996). The identifi cation and validation of distinct depressive syndromes in a population-based sample of female twins. *Archives of General Psychiatry*, 53 , 391 – 399.

Lakka HM, Laaksonen DE, Lakka TA, Niskanen LK, Kumpusalo E, Tuomilehto J, Salonen JT (2002). The metabolic syndrome and total and cardiovascular disease mortality in middle-aged men. *JAMA* 288, 2709–2716.

Merikangas, K. R., He, J. P., Burstein, M., Swanson, S. A., Avenevoli, S., Cui, L., Swendsen, J (2010). Lifetime prevalence of mental disorders in US adolescents: Results from the national comorbidity survey replication–adolescent supplement (NCS-A). *Journal of the American Academy of Child and Adolescent Psychiatry*, 49, 980–989. doi:10.1016/ j.jaac. 2010. 05.017.

Must A, Strauss RS (1999). Risks and consequences of childhood and adolescent obesity, *Int. J. Obes. Relat. Metab. Disord.* Suppl 2:S2-11.

Olfson M (2012). Epidemiologic and clinical perspectives on antipsychotic treatment of children and adolescents. *Can. J. Psychiatry*. 2012 Dec;57 (12):715-6.

Panagiotopoulos C, Ronsley R, Kuzeljevic B, Davidson J (2012). Waist circumference is a sensitive screening tool for assessment of metabolic syndrome risk in children treated with second- generation antipsychotics. *Can. J. Psychiatry*. 2012 Jan; 57(1):34-44.

Räikkönen K, Matthews KA, Kuller LH (2007). Depressive symptoms *Diabetes Care*. 30, 872-877.

Scheimann AO (2012). Overview of paediatric obesity for the paediatric mental health provider. *International Review of Psychiatry*; 24(3): 231–240.

Spear, B. A., Barlow, S. E., Ervin, C., Ludwig, D. S., Saelens, B. E., Schetzina, K. E. & Taveras, E.M (2007). Recommendations for treatment of child and adolescent overweight and obesity. *Pediatrics*, 120, S254–88. doi:10.1542/peds. 2007 - 2329F.

Wang Y, Lim H (2012). The global childhood *Int. Rev. Psychiatry.* 2012 Jun;24(3):176-88.

Waring, M. E. & Lapane, K. L (2008). Overweight in children and adolescents in relation to attention-defi cit/hyperactivity disorder: results from a national sample. *Pediatrics*, 122, e1 – 6.

WHO (2010). Childhood overweight and obesity. http://www.who.int/ dietphysicalactivity/childhood/en/

Wolkoff LE, Tanofsky-Kraff M, Shomaker LB, Kozlosky M, Columbo KM, Elliott CA, Ranzenhofer LM, Osborn RL, Yanovski SZ, Yanovski JA (2011). *Eat. Behav.*; 12(1):15-20. doi: 10.1016/j.eatbeh.2010.09.001. Epub 2010 Sep 18.

INDEX

T

U